# The
# Black
# Book
# on
# Canadian
# Medical
# Schools

Dr. Brett L. Ferdinand, MD
(author of The Gold Standard MCAT text)
with
Mia Lalonde, LL B

# www.MCAT-prep.com
**The *only* prep you need™.**

RuveneCo
Inc

# The Black Book on Canadian Medical Schools

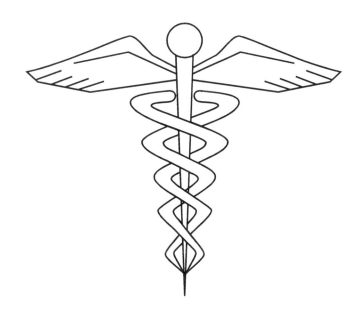

## Authors

Brett L. Ferdinand BSc MD-CM FRCSC
Mia Lalonde BA LL B

## Marketing Manager

Janice Fijalkowski BComm

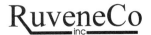

RuveneCo
inc

Address all inquiries, comments, or suggestions to the publisher:

E-mail: ruveneco@bellnet.ca
Web: www.ruveneco.com

RuveneCo Inc., Publications
1641 Place Victor Hugo
Montreal, QC  H3C-4P3

ISBN: 0-9730806-2-0

Printed in Canada.

# About the Chief Author

During his undergraduate career at the University of Ottawa, Dr. Ferdinand was awarded numerous scholarships *en route* to graduating with honors in a B.Sc. program in 1989. More than ten years ago, confident that he would one day be a doctor, the undergraduate student Brett Ferdinand fulfilled his love for teaching by creating *The Medical School Preparatory Course* (MSPC™), which has become a perennial lecture series. The course was the first to teach both the MCAT and the details of the admissions process and now is also available online (www.MCAT-prep.com). There are many practising Canadian physicians who attended his lectures in the early years.

After excelling at the MCAT, he was accepted by all the medical schools to which he applied. During medical school at McGill he continued to teach and then completed the MCAT text: *The Gold Standard for Medical School Admissions*. The book received distribution throughout North America and instantly became one of the best selling MCAT manuals in Canada. The text, now at over 1000 pages, has entered its $10^{th}$ year and continues to stand as the flagship for the industry. He had also produced, new for the year 2000 and beyond, *The Silver Bullet: Real MCATs Explained*.

Dr. Ferdinand graduated from medical school in 1993 and completed residency training in General and Trauma Surgery. Over the past few years, he has performed surgery in Quebec, Ontario and Manitoba. He continues to give lectures on the admissions process, on the basic sciences for the MCAT, and is well known as a dynamic lecturer who makes difficult concepts easy to understand. Over the years he has lectured to thousands of pre-medical students and reached thousands more through his books. He is pursuing a career active in teaching, basic science research and general surgery.

# PREFACE

The first 10 chapters of this book are mostly based on experience. Some of the material was used with permission from *The Gold Standard* and then altered for the Canadian context. Names were altered in sample interviews, autobiographical materials and the letter of reference to protect the identities of those who volunteered to have the information published.

The last two chapters, which cover the medical schools, are mostly based on research. Printed material from the medical schools were reviewed. Subsequently, all 16 Canadian medical schools were provided with questionnaires to give an opportunity for deans, assistant deans and admissions officers to provide more insight into their programs. Telephone and/or personal interviews were conducted when necessary to clarify specific aspects of admissions. Most of the medical schools were very cooperative and we give our sincere thanks.

Rankings of the medical schools are based on the American-based evaluation called: The Gourman Report. It is published by National Education Standards and it is the most internationally recognized ratings book. It is available at most university libraries. Though all Canadian schools are viewed highly by the report, many are not pleased by being ranked nor by the criteria used. Some of the arguments are valid; however, this book is written for the benefit of pre-medical students and the fact that they are also ranked by criteria they cannot influence tipped the scale for me to include the rankings!

Information regarding US medical schools was acquired by logging on to the web site of the individual medical schools. Most of these sites are extremely informative and Chapter 9 will show you how to gain access. Unknowns were determined using telephone interviews and with information from pre-medical web sites. Most of the information was consistent with Medical School Admissions Requirements, published by the Association of American Medical Colleges (an authorized resource), and a similar annual review by US News & World Report. Students who require more information with respect to US medical schools should refer to these publications.

A special thanks goes out to Mia Lalonde. Much of the research was accomplished by the drive, creativity and intellect of Miss Lalonde. There is hardly a better example of self-directed learning than a law student studying admissions to medical school. She is now beginning her law practice. Her future is certainly bright.

Much gratitude also goes out to Bradley Dottin. He is a chemist extraordinaire, a computer wizard and most importantly, a friend. Thanks also to My Linh Lam who contributed updates to an earlier edition.

This book is, wholeheartedly, dedicated to our parents.

# Table of Contents

# INTRODUCTION

We have now entered the 21st century. The innumerable developments which have occurred in the last one hundred years have forever affected the delivery of health-care in our country. Medical schools have equally evolved but the changes have been punctuated over the last 30 years. Acceptance to medical schools based exclusively on grades is now frowned upon by both the academic medical community as well as society in general. Pre-requisites strictly based on the four classic pre-medical sciences (biology, physics, general and organic chemistry) have been replaced, for the most part, by either requiring a broader based pre-medical education or by not requiring any specific courses in order to encourage exploration.

With the immense competition to become accepted to a Canadian medical school, combined with the flux in the system and an unhealthy fixation on rumours, candidates have become cynical. Many believe that the admissions process is based on randomness, bias, luck or worse - contacts. Though there may be an element of truth in every lie, the rule has been clouded by a smoke screen: there is no magic to medical school admissions.

Students have difficulty understanding how their friend with an A- average, "tons of volunteer work and a really nice person," is not accepted to medical school, while the B+ student who is "just OK," is accepted. The answer is simple: great candidates may have mediocre applications, and vice versa. Speaking from experience, the student who prepares for the admissions process can pick the school and the date for their admission. This is not arrogance, it is a belief that the system works and when you have more that just fulfilled the stated needs of the medical school, the great likelihood is that you will be accepted.

Confidence begins by understanding the admissions process. Read about the different medical schools which interest you. Write to them. Clarify any outstanding issues. Note the difference in importance placed on academic aspects like GPA or MCAT results or on non-academic aspects like letters of reference, autobiographical materials or interviews. Be sure you are aware of the regional and/or provincial considerations.

When you know the grades and/or MCAT scores you need - prepare, study, attain your goals with some to spare. Along the route, bend your thoughts to the non-academic part of the application: prepare, learn, read, and practice. All these things you do as if your future career depends on it, because it does. It is possible for the unprepared charismatic student to be accepted to medical school. Do not let the exception become the rule.

This book is unique. It is designed to address the entire admissions process to a Canadian medical school. We begin by discussing your choice of undergraduate studies and how to improve your grades (Chapter 1). We then look at the application services and how you convert your grades to scales used by some medical schools (Chapter 2). The MCAT is then dissected, necessary scores discussed and a clear plan to excel is presented (Chapters 3 and 4). Then we turn to the non-academic aspect of admissions. The interview is explored followed by sample questions and answers (Chapters 5 and 6). A discussion on autobiographical materials and letters of reference are each followed by sample successful submissions (Chapters 7 and 8). The next chapter presents some nice information regarding how the internet can help you (Chapter 9). An important chapter to give you the proper historical context to the current changes and trends in medical school admissions and education is Chapter 10.

Of course, the *sine qua non* of the book is Chapter 11. All Canadian medical schools are presented from East to West (as of 2005, there are 17). Included in the reviews are the relevant addresses, requirements, deadlines, rankings, etc. Where possible, GPA and MCAT scores and the formula used in the admissions process are revealed. The latter is a lot like the proverbial picture, it is worth a thousand words.

Some translations may be helpful. A "cutoff" means if you scored lower, you will not be accepted. Some schools, however, will take exceptional circumstances into consideration for students below the cutoff. A "flag" means that if you have met that requirement then that requirement is no longer an issue in the admissions process. Thus scoring much above the "flag" does not help your admissions chances, but scoring below eliminates your application from further processing. Warning: many medical schools are no longer including the current year of studies in their calculations for cutoffs. "A minimum grade/MCAT of X is expected" is translated as neither a cutoff nor a flag. Rather it sets a standard but leaves the door open. Average scores provide a lot of information about the emphasis of a program, and along with the minimum score, provides students with a good idea of how they compare to what they need for admissions.

And finally, the US option is explored in Chapter 12 which includes the names and addresses of the more than 100 US medical schools with recent GPA and MCAT averages of students admitted to their programs. In the Appendix, you will find The Hippocratic Oath and information about materials to help you prepare for the MCAT.

The admissions process is imperfect and as such will continue to undergo change. The objective of this book is simple: to underline the fact that the greatest factor affecting your chances of being accepted to medical school is you. The quality of your application does not depend on anyone else. There is no perfect candidate but you must strive to excel in the various aspects of the application. There are more than 1500 positions in Canadian medical schools available each year. There is enough room for both sexes, all religions, all races and for great diversity in culture and experience. Use your unique experiences to clarify your decision to pursue medicine as a career. Once this is done, buckle up and get ready for the ride... By the way, you're driving.

# Medical School Admissions

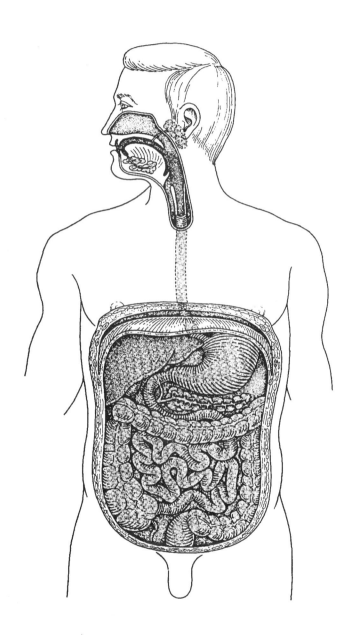

# Chapter 1
# ACADEMIC SUCCESS

*A little learning is a dangerous thing;*
*Drink deep, or taste not the Pierian spring;*
*There shallow draughts intoxicate the brain,*
*And drinking largely sobers us again.*

**Alexander Pope**, Essay on Criticism

## Choosing a Course of Study

One of the greatest aspects of current admission requirements to medical schools is the liberty given to students in choosing a course of study. The university student completing an undergraduate degree in economics, biology, languages or psychology, all essentially have the same opportunity for admissions. The importance of this concept cannot be overstated. Every year many students are herded into programs like biochemistry and physiology, not for the love of the program, but rather because of fantasies of an improved chance of admissions to medical studies. The fabrication worsens as students rationalize their choices on the basis that when they take similar courses in medical school, they will perform better.

A few clarifications are in order. To begin with, the person who performs best in anatomy in medical school tends to be the student who never had studied anatomy as an undergraduate student. While the medical student with the major in anatomy is concentrating elsewhere, the novice is learning at an exponential rate. Previous experience is not necessarily well correlated with future success. Secondly, the aspect of your undergraduate record which has the *greater* impact on all Canadian medical schools, bar none, is the grade *not* the course of study.

If you love biochemistry then please pursue it. If architecture, business or physics is more to your liking, stretch your mind and explore. The key is to choose a course of study and/or electives which you enjoy. Consequently, the likelihood is strongest that you will perform optimally. This is the beauty of the admissions process - to broaden your scope of experience is not simply acceptable, it is laudable.

## Academic Coherence

As a rule, it will work to your advantage to maintain yourself as a full-time student (since the definition of 'full-time' varies among medical schools clarify ambiguities in advance of course selection; part-time students must clarify the conditions of eligibility with individual medical schools). It is also important to have completed the expected number of credits during the prescribed time period, even if this necessitates completing summer courses.  A few medical schools, however, will accept credits received for summer courses but will not include the grade into the overall grade point average (GPA) for admissions.

Academic coherence must be evident in your course of study.  If the logic of your course selection is not evident then you must address the issue in your autobiographical materials or during the medical school interview.  Do not apologize for taking a particular course of study, rather, describe the characteristics you learnt or developed which may be relevant to the study of medicine.

Carefully analyse the pre-requisites for the medical schools which interest you.  It is critical that you spend time to ensure that you have fulfilled all the basic academic requirements.  As a rule, the year of your academic program should generally correspond to the "year" of your courses.  If the preceding is not the case then provide good reasons.

It's OK to be different, everybody is!  Most students think that their academic history is unique.  Well, at this very moment, there are students studying medicine who had taken time off from school, who had had a horrible undergraduate year, who changed undergraduate programs, who had to re-write the MCAT, who completed a PhD, who completed two bachelor degrees, who are over 40 years old, etc.  Medical schools have even designed their admissions requirements to allow for the enormous diversity in the applicant pool.  The message is simple.  Be sure you are pursuing a course of study in which, each day, you can look forward to attending the lectures.

## Lectures

Before you set foot in a classroom you should consider the value of being there.  Even if you were taking a course like 'Basket-weaving 101,' one way to help you do well in the course is to consider the value of the course to **you**.  The course should have an *intrinsic* value (i.e. 'I enjoy weaving baskets').  The course will also have an *extrinsic* value (i.e. 'If I do not get good grades, I will not be accepted...').  Motivation, a positive attitude, and an interest in learning give you an edge before the class even begins.

Unless there is a student 'note-taking club' for your courses, your attendance record and the quality of your notes should both be as excellent as possible.  Be sure to choose seating in the classroom which ensures that you will be able to hear the professor adequately and see whatever she may write.  Whenever possible, do not sit close to friends!

Instead of chattering before the lecture begins, spend the idle moments quickly reviewing the previous lecture in that subject so you would have an idea of what to expect.  Try to take good notes and pay close attention.  The preceding may sound like a difficult combination (esp. with professors who speak and write quickly); however, with practice you can learn to do it well.

And finally, do not let the quality of teaching affect your interest in the subject nor your grades! Do not waste your time during or before lectures complaining about how the professor speaks too quickly, does not explain concepts adequately, etc... When the time comes, you can mention such issues on the appropriate evaluation forms! In the meantime, consider this: despite the good or poor quality of teaching, there is always a certain number of students who **still** perform well. You must strive to count yourself among those students.

## Taking Notes

Unless your professor says otherwise, if you take excellent notes and learn them inside out, you will *ace* his course. Your notes should always be up-to-date, complete, and separate from other subjects.

To be safe, you should try to write everything! You can fill in any gaps by comparing your notes with those of your friends. You can create your own shorthand symbols or use standard ones. The following represents some useful symbols:

| | | | |
|---|---|---|---|
| \|•\| | *between* | $\bar{c}$ or w | *with* |
| = | *the same as* | $\bar{c}$out or w/o | *without* |
| ≠ | *not the same as* | esp. | *especially* |
| ∴ | *therefore* | ∵ | *because* |
| cf. | *compare* | i.e. | *that is* |
| Δ | *difference, change in* | e.g. | *for example* |

Many students rewrite their notes at home. Should you decide to rewrite your notes, your time will be used efficiently if you are paying close attention to the information you are rewriting. In fact, a more useful technique is the following: during class, write your notes only on the right side of your binder. Later, rewrite the information from class in a complete but condensed form on the left side of the binder (*this condensed form should include* **mnemonics** *which we will discuss later*).

Some students find it valuable to use different colour pens. Juggling pens in class may distract you from the content of the lecture. Different colour pens would be more useful in the context of rewriting one's notes.

## The Principles of Studying Efficiently

If you study efficiently, you will have enough time for extracurricular activities, movies, etc. The bottom line is that your time must be used efficiently and effectively.

During the average school day, time can be found during breaks, between classes, and after school to quickly review notes in a library or any other quiet place you can find on campus. Simply by using the available time in your school day, you can keep up to date with recent information.

You should design a personal study schedule to meet your particular needs. However, as a rule, a certain amount of time every evening should be set aside for more in depth studying. Week-ends can be set aside for special projects and reviewing notes from the beginning.

On the surface, the idea of regularly reviewing notes from the beginning may sound like an insurmountable task which would take forever! The reality is just the opposite. After all, if you continually study the information, by the time mid-terms approach you would have seen the first lecture so many times that it would take only moments to review it again. On the other hand, had you not been reviewing regularly, it would be like reading that lecture for the first time!

You should study wherever you are comfortable and effective studying (i.e. library, at home, etc.). Should you prefer studying at home, be sure to create an environment which is conducive to studying.

Studying should be an active process to memorize and understand a given set of material. Memorization and comprehension are best achieved by the **elaboration** of course material, **attention**, **repetition**, and practising **retrieval** of the information. All these principles are borne out in the following techniques.

## Studying from Notes and Texts

Successful studying from either class notes or textbooks can be accomplished in three simple steps:

* **Preview the material**: read all the relevant headings, titles, and sub-titles to give you a general idea of what you are about to learn. You should never embark on a trip without knowing where you are going!

* **Read while questioning**: passive studying is when you sit in front of a book and just read. This can lead to boredom, lack of concentration, or even worse - difficulty remembering what you just read! Active studying involves reading while actively questioning yourself. For example: how does this fit in with the `big picture'? How does this relate to what we learned last week? What cues about these words or lists will make it easy for me to memorize them? What type of question would my professor ask me? If I was asked a question on this material, how would I answer? Etc...

* **Recite and consider**: put the notes or text away while you attempt to recall the main facts. Once you are able to recite the important information, consider how it relates to the entire subject.

N.B. if you ever sit down to study and you are not quite sure with which subject to begin, always start with either the most difficult subject or the subject you like least (usually they are one in the same!).

## Study Aids

The most effective study aids include practice exams, mnemonics and audio cassettes.

**Practice exams** (*exams from previous semesters*) are often available from the library, upper level students, or sometimes from the professor. They can be used like maps which guide you through your semester. They give you a good indication as to what information you should emphasize when you study; what question types and exam format you can expect; and what your level of progress is.

One practice exam should be set aside to write one week before `the real thing'. You should time yourself and write the exam in an environment free from distractions. This provides an ideal way to uncover unexpected weak points.

**Mnemonics** are an effective way of memorizing lists of information. Usually a word, phrase, or sentence is constructed to symbolize a greater amount of information (i.e. LEO is A GERC = Lose Electrons is Oxidation is Anode, Gain Electrons is Reduction at Cathode). An effective study aid to active studying is the creation of your own mnemonics.

**Audio cassettes** can be used as effective tools to repeat information and to use your time efficiently. Information from the left side of your notes (*see Taking Notes*) including mnemonics, can be dictated onto cassette. Often, an entire semester of work can be summarized into one 90 minute cassette.

Now you can listen to the cassettes in a walkman while waiting in line at the bank, or in a bus or with a car stereo on the way to school, work, etc. You can also listen to a cassette when you go to sleep and listen to another one first thing in the morning. You are probably familiar with the situation of having heard a song early in the morning and then having difficulty, for the rest of the day, getting it out of your mind! Well, imagine if the first thing you heard in the morning was: "Hair is a modified keratinized structure produced by the cylindrical downgrowth of epithelium...". Thus the cassette becomes an effective study aid since it is an extra source of repetition.

Some students like to **tape lectures**. Though it may be helpful to fill in missing notes, it is not an efficient way to repeat information.

Some students like to use **study cards** on which they may write either a summary of information they must memorize or relevant questions to consider. Then the cards are used throughout the day to quickly flash information to promote thought on course material.

## Falling Behind

Imagine yourself as a marathon runner who has run 25.5 km of a 26 km race. The finishing line is now in view. However, you have fallen behind some of the other runners. The most difficult aspect of the race is still ahead.

In such a scenario some interesting questions can be asked: Is now the time to drop out of the race because 0.5 km suddenly seems like a long distance? Is now the time to reevaluate whether or not you should have competed? Or is now the time to remain faithful to your goals and give 100%?

Imagine one morning in mid-semester you wake up realizing you have fallen behind in your studies. What do you do? Where do you start? Is it too late?

Like a doctor being presented with an urgent matter, you should see the situation as one of life's challenges. Now is the worst time for doubts, rather, it is the time for action. A clear line of action should be formulated such that it could be followed.

For example, one might begin by gathering all pertinent study materials like a complete set of study notes, relevant text(s), sample exams, etc. As a rule, to get back into the thick of things, notes and sample exams take precedence. Studying at this point should take a three-pronged approach: i) a regular, consistent review of the information from your notes from the beginning of the section for which you are responsible (i.e. *starting with the first class*); ii) a regular, consistent review of course material as you are learning it from the lectures (*this is the most efficient way to study*); iii) regular testing using questions given in class or those contained in sample exams. Using such questions will clarify the extent of your progress.

It is also of value, as time allows, to engage in extracurricular activities which you find helpful in reducing stress (i.e. sports, piano, creative writing, etc.).

# Chapter 2

# APPLICATION SERVICES AND CONVERTING GRADES

---

*Medicine . . . the only profession that labours incessantly to destroy the reason for its own existence.*

**Sir James Bryce**, Address - 23 March, 1914

## Overview

The ideal way to get an adequate amount of information about medical schools and their admission policies is to call or write the individual medical schools to which you would like to apply. Subsequently, they may send you letters responding to your questions, pamphlets or other documents which will enlighten your knowledge of each specific school.

If it is important to you how a medical school rates worldwide, you can consult the *Gourman Report* which is available at most large university libraries. Special editions of the *U.S. News and World Report* and *Maclean's Magazine* also rate university programs. If you want statistical information on the medical schools and admissions in the United States and Canada, the latest edition of *Medical School Admission Requirements* may be helpful. It is available from the AAMC (*see Chapter 3 for the address*). The Association of Canadian Medical Colleges, based in Ottawa, publishes a manual every two years reviewing statistical information, admission requirements and selection policies of Canadian medical schools.

## Application Services

Application services for the admissions process help to filter and standardize information for the participating medical schools. Application services do not render admission decisions; rather, they provide a processing service. In the U.S., approximately 110 of the 126 medical schools participate in the American Medical College Application Service (AMCAS). AMCAS application materials may be obtained from premedical advisors, participating medical schools or you may write:

AMCAS, Section for Student Services
Association of American Medical Colleges
2450 N Street, N.W., Suite 201
Washington, D.C. 20037-1131

# APPLICATION SERVICES

Phone: (202) 828-0600
Web: www.aamc.org

There is also an application service in Canada. However, eleven of the sixteen Canadian medical schools have individualized application procedures. The five medical schools in the Province of Ontario participate in the Ontario Medical School Application Service (OMSAS). OMSAS application materials may be obtained from participating medical schools or you may write:

OMSAS
P.O. Box 1328
650 Woodlawn Rd. West
Guelph, Ontario
Canada, N1H 7P4
(519) 823-1940
E-mail: omsas@ouac.on.ca
Web: www.ouac.on.ca

Some medical schools in the US that participate in application services may *also* have their own applications to fill out. Thus despite the existence of application services, nothing can replace the importance of contacting specific medical schools to be informed about their programs, policies, tuition, admission requirements, application procedures, etc. For any medical school that may interest you, *as early as possible* you should write and clarify, among other issues, their application procedures.

## Converting Grades

OMSAS has engineered a table which allows students to convert grades from their university to the GPA out of 4.0 used in the admissions process. The same scale is used for all the Ontario medical schools. The University of Alberta, which has a 9.0 scale, uses the same conversion table though it is clearly not a member of OMSAS.

Full-year courses receive a weight of 2, half-year or semester courses receive a weight of 1, a quarter course gets .7, and a separately graded lab course gets a weight of one half of the preceding values. Calculate by multiplying the converted grade by the course length. Add total OMSAS values and divide by total course lengths to supply you with your final converted average out of 4.0. Now you can estimate your scores and compare them with the requirements you will find in the following chapters. Use the scale listed next to the name of your university. If your school uses letter grades only, then use Scale 7.

## University Programs

Alberta 1
Athabasca 3
Bishop's 3
British Columbia 5, 7
Brock 3
Cape Breton 3
Carleton 7
Guelph 3
Lakehead 3
Laurentian/Laurentienne 3
McGill 6, 7
McMaster 7
Memorial 6
Mt. Allison 3, 7
Mt. Saint Vincent 5
Nipissing 3
Ottawa 7
Prince Edward Island 3
Queen's 3
Regina 3
Royal Military College 3, 7
Ryerson 7
Sainte-Anne 3
Saskatchewan 3
St. Francis Xavier 3
Technical U. of Nova Scotia 3
Toronto 3, 7
Trent 3
Waterloo 3, 7
Western Ontario 3
Wilfrid Laurier 7
Windsor 7
York 3, 7

## Conversion Table (OMSAS)

| Scale 1 | | Scale 2 | | Scale 3 | | Scale 4 | | Scale 5 | | Scale 6 | | Scale 7 | |
|---|---|---|---|---|---|---|---|---|---|---|---|---|---|
| 9 | 4.00 | 8 | 4.00 | 100 | 4.00 | 100 | 4.00 | 100 | 4.00 | 100 | 4.00 | A+ | 4.00 |
| | | | | 99 | 4.00 | 99 | 4.00 | 99 | 4.00 | 99 | 4.00 | | |
| | | | | 98 | 4.00 | 98 | 4.00 | 98 | 4.00 | 98 | 4.00 | | |
| | | | | 97 | 4.00 | 97 | 4.00 | 97 | 4.00 | 97 | 4.00 | | |
| | | | | 96 | 4.00 | 96 | 4.00 | 96 | 4.00 | 96 | 4.00 | | |
| | | | | 95 | 4.00 | 95 | 4.00 | 95 | 4.00 | 95 | 4.00 | | |
| | | | | 94 | 4.00 | 94 | 4.00 | 94 | 4.00 | 94 | 4.00 | | |
| | | | | 93 | 4.00 | 93 | 3.98 | 93 | 3.98 | 93 | 3.98 | | |
| | | | | 92 | 4.00 | 92 | 3.98 | 92 | 3.95 | 92 | 3.96 | | |
| | | | | 91 | 4.00 | 91 | 3.96 | 91 | 3.93 | 91 | 3.94 | | |
| | | | | 90 | 4.00 | 90 | 3.94 | 90 | 3.90 | 90 | 3.92 | | |
| | | | | 89 | 3.97 | 89 | 3.92 | 89 | 3.87 | 89 | 3.90 | | |
| | | | | 88 | 3.93 | 88 | 3.90 | 88 | 3.85 | 88 | 3.88 | | |
| | | | | 87 | 3.90 | 87 | 3.88 | 87 | 3.82 | 87 | 3.86 | A | 3.90 |
| | | | | 86 | 3.87 | 86 | 3.86 | 86 | 3.79 | 86 | 3.82 | | |
| | | | | 85 | 3.83 | 85 | 3.84 | 85 | 3.76 | 85 | 3.80 | | |
| | | | | 84 | 3.79 | 84 | 3.82 | 84 | 3.73 | 84 | 3.77 | | |
| | | | | 83 | 3.75 | 83 | 3.80 | 83 | 3.70 | 83 | 3.73 | | |
| 8 | 3.70 | 7 | 3.70 | 82 | 3.70 | 82 | 3.77 | 82 | 3.67 | 82 | 3.70 | A- | 3.70 |
| | | | | 81 | 3.65 | 81 | 3.75 | 81 | 3.64 | 81 | 3.67 | | |
| | | | | 80 | 3.61 | 80 | 3.72 | 80 | 3.61 | 80 | 3.63 | | |
| | | | | 79 | 3.50 | 79 | 3.70 | 79 | 3.50 | 79 | 3.52 | | |
| | | | | 78 | 3.40 | 78 | 3.68 | 78 | 3.40 | 78 | 3.41 | | |
| 7 | 3.30 | 6 | 3.30 | 77 | 3.30 | 77 | 3.65 | 77 | 3.30 | 77 | 3.30 | B+ | 3.30 |
| | | | | 76 | 3.20 | 76 | 3.63 | 76 | 3.20 | 76 | 3.19 | | |
| | | | | 75 | 3.10 | 75 | 3.60 | 75 | 3.10 | 75 | 3.08 | | |
| | | | | 74 | 3.00 | 74 | 3.45 | 74 | 3.07 | 74 | 3.06 | B | 3.0 |
| | | | | 73 | 2.90 | 73 | 3.30 | 73 | 3.03 | 73 | 3.03 | | |
| | | | | 72 | 2.80 | 72 | 3.15 | 72 | 3.00 | 72 | 3.00 | | |
| 6 | 2.70 | 5 | 2.70 | 71 | 2.70 | 71 | 3.08 | 71 | 2.97 | 71 | 2.97 | B- | 2.70 |
| | | | | 70 | 2.60 | 70 | 3.00 | 70 | 2.93 | 70 | 2.94 | | |
| | | | | 69 | 2.50 | 69 | 2.92 | 69 | 2.86 | 69 | 2.86 | | |
| | | | | 68 | 2.40 | 68 | 2.81 | 68 | 2.78 | 68 | 2.78 | | |
| 5 | 2.30 | 4 | 2.30 | 67 | 2.30 | 67 | 2.70 | 67 | 2.70 | 67 | 2.70 | C+ | 2.30 |
| | | | | 66 | 2.20 | 66 | 2.59 | 66 | 2.62 | 66 | 2.62 | | |
| | | | | 65 | 2.10 | 65 | 2.45 | 65 | 2.54 | 65 | 2.54 | | |
| | | | | 64 | 2.00 | 64 | 2.15 | 64 | 2.46 | 64 | 2.46 | C | 2.00 |
| | | | | 63 | 1.90 | 63 | 2.05 | 63 | 2.38 | 63 | 2.38 | | |
| | | | | 62 | 1.80 | 62 | 1.95 | 62 | 2.30 | 62 | 2.30 | | |
| 4 | 1.70 | 3 | 1.70 | 61 | 1.70 | 61 | 1.80 | 61 | 2.22 | 61 | 2.22 | C- | 1.70 |
| | | | | 60 | 1.60 | 60 | 1.60 | 60 | 2.14 | 60 | 2.14 | | |
| | | | | 59 | 1.50 | 59 | 1.45 | 59 | 2.10 | 59 | 2.10 | | |
| | | | | 58 | 1.40 | 58 | 1.35 | 58 | 2.05 | 58 | 2.05 | | |
| | | 2 | 1.30 | 57 | 1.30 | 57 | 1.25 | 57 | 2.00 | 57 | 2.00 | D+ | 1.30 |
| | | | | 56 | 1.20 | 56 | 1.15 | 56 | 1.95 | 56 | 1.95 | | |
| | | | | 55 | 1.10 | 55 | 1.10 | 55 | 1.90 | 55 | 1.90 | | |
| | | | | 54 | 1.00 | 54 | 1.00 | 54 | 1.84 | 54 | 1.60 | D | 1.00 |
| | | | | 53 | 0.09 | 53 | 0.90 | 53 | 1.77 | 53 | 1.30 | | |
| | | | | 52 | 0.08 | 52 | 0.80 | 52 | 1.70 | 52 | 1.00 | | |
| | | | | 51 | 0.07 | 51 | 0.70 | 51 | 1.63 | 51 | 0.70 | D- | 0.70 |
| | | | | 50 | 0.06 | 50 | 0.60 | 50 | 1.56 | 50 | 0.40 | | |

# Chapter 3

# THE STRUCTURE OF THE *new* MCAT

---

*All interest in disease and death is only another expression of interest in life.*

**Thomas Mann**, The Magic Mountain

## Introduction

The *new* Medical College Admission Test (MCAT) is a prerequisite for admission to nearly all the medical schools in North America. Each year, over 40,000 applicants to American and Canadian medical schools submit MCAT test results. While the actual weight given to MCAT scores in the admissions process varies from school to school, often they are regarded in a similar manner to your college/university CGPA (i.e. your academic standing).

In applying to some medical schools, for example, the MCAT score is as important as all of your years of undergraduate study! On the other hand, some universities will set a minimum level of performance on the MCAT and then analyse school grades to decide who will be invited to the interviews. In this context, the MCAT is the Great Equalizer. Acing the MCAT makes you a star no matter how poorly *Maclean's Magazine* rates your undergraduate program! Furthermore, if a student receives a "D" in a first year physics course, there is hardly a better remedy than to ace the Physical Sciences section of the MCAT. Any way you look at it, doing well is imperative for most applicants.

Further evidence for the equalizing power of the MCAT is the following: medical schools which rely exclusively on grades to decide who gets interviewed, have the highest academic averages needed for admissions in that region. Medical schools that decide based on the highest combined GPA/MCAT scores have lower average GPAs but higher average MCAT scores. There is no coincidence since some students are making up for a lower GPA by doing well on the MCAT.

The MCAT is required by all Canadian medical schools except: (1) the French language medical schools in Quebec, though Université Laval will consider MCAT scores if submitted; (2) University of Ottawa (Canada's only bilingual medical school); (3) McMaster University; and (4) the Northern Ontario Medical School.

Research has suggested that the MCAT has a positive predictive value. It appears that MCAT scores are a slightly better predictor of first year medical school grades than are undergraduate GPAs (*Academic Medicine*, Vol 69 (5), p. 394-400, May 1994). Further research is ongoing.

The MCAT is administered on a Saturday biannually, before the beginning of the academic year (August) and at the end of the academic year (April). To register for the MCAT, you should consult your undergraduate adviser or write to:

---

# THE STRUCTURE OF THE *new* MCAT

MCAT Program
P.O. Box 4056
Iowa City, Iowa, 52243
Phone: (319) 337-1357; www.aamc.org

Most medical schools require that you would have written the MCAT by the Fall of the year preceding the projected date of admissions. However, some medical schools will permit you to *re-write* the MCAT in the April preceding admissions.

## The Format of the *new* MCAT

The MCAT will not only test your scientific knowledge in biology, physics, inorganic and organic chemistry, but will also measure your problem-solving, critical thinking and writing skills. The exam is divided into four sections. All questions, save the Writing Sample, are multiple choice with four choices per question.

The MCAT is over seven hours long (including breaks). There are two morning sections and two afternoon sections separated by a lunch break. This is the schedule for the test day:

| | |
|---|---|
| Physical Sciences: | 100 minutes |
| Break: | (10 minutes) |
| | |
| Verbal Reasoning: | 85 minutes |
| Lunch: | (60 minutes) |
| | |
| Writing Sample: | 60 minutes |
| Break: | (10 minutes) |

Biological Sciences: 100 minutes

## How the MCAT is Scored

The MCAT is scored for each of the four sections individually. The sections consisting of multiple choice questions are first scored right or wrong resulting in a raw score. Note that wrong answers are worth the same as unanswered questions so ALWAYS ANSWER ALL THE QUESTIONS even if you are not sure of certain answers. The raw score is then converted to a scaled score ranging from 1 (lowest) to 15 (highest). The scores are scaled to ensure that the same proportion of individual marks within each section (i.e. 1-15) are given year to year.

The essay is scored by two readers on a scale of 1 (lowest) to 6 (highest). The combined scores from the two readers are then converted to a scale ranging from J (lowest) to T (highest). To illustrate, the following are the letter grades with the resulting combined scores in brackets: J (2), K (3), L (4), M (5), N (6), O (7), P (8), Q (9), R (10), S (11), and T (12).

The scores for each section are reported to you, the schools you designate and, with your permission, to your undergraduate advisor. Generally, your results are valid from 2 to 5 years from the time you wrote the exam, depending on the medical school.

As you will come to learn in the following chapters, most medical schools require a minimum score of 8 on any given multiple choice section. The average scores of students admitted to Canadian medical schools tends to be between 10 and 11 in the multiple choice sections, and between N and Q in the Writing Sample. The weight the MCAT has on your chances of admissions varies greatly from one medical school to another.

Every MCAT includes a small number of questions which will not be scored. These questions are either used to calibrate the exam or were found to be either too ambiguous or too difficult to be counted. So if you see a question that you think is off the wall, unanswerable or inappropriate, it could well be one of these questions so never panic!

## The *new* MCAT: A Closer Look

### Physical Sciences (100 minutes)

This section is made up of 77 multiple choice questions divided half and half between general chemistry and physics. Questions in groups of 4 to 8, based on a 250-word passage will account for 62 of the questions. The remaining 15 questions will be independent of one another and of any passage. All the questions test your knowledge and understanding of concepts and your scientific problem-solving skills in chemistry and physics. You are not expected to memorize extensive amounts of material for this section of the MCAT.

An important part of the Physical Sciences section is the testing of your ability to read data presented in tabular and in graphical forms. You should therefore be familiar with the basic principles used in the presentation of data. You should also be able to identify trends and tendencies, as well as relationships in the data presented. Furthermore, you may be asked to identify the best way of presenting a particular set of data.

The concepts in chemistry and physics tested on the MCAT are those generally taught in introductory level college/university courses. While the passages may present advanced concepts, the questions accompanying the passage will only require a knowledge of basic principles. Thus, more advanced chemistry and physics courses are not required for this test. You should know the constants and formulae associated with elementary work as presented in this manual and listed in the AAMC manuals. Other equations and constants will be provided in the actual MCAT exam, along with a periodic table of the elements. Finally, some basic mathematical knowledge is expected as calculators are <u>not allowed</u> for this test.

### Mathematics Needed for the MCAT

For the MCAT you should:

1>      Be able to perform arithmetic calculations such as additions, subtractions, multiplications and divisions as well as be able to use proportions, percentages, ratios and estimations of square roots. If you have difficulty with basic arithmetic, you should include time in your review to practice. For the MCAT, you must be <u>accurate and quick</u>.

2>    Be familiar with metric units and how to convert between metric and imperial units using given conversion factors. Know how to balance equations containing physical units.

3>    Understand logarithms, scientific notation, quadratic and simultaneous equations, and graphical representations of data in various scales at the level of advanced high school algebra.

4>    Know how to calculate an arithmetic mean and to determine the range for a given set of data. An understanding of the general concepts associated with statistics (correlation, association, etc.) is expected, but no calculations of standard deviations and correlation coefficients are required.

5>    Be able to calculate at an elementary level the mathematical probability of an event.

6>    Be familiar with the basic concepts of trigonometry and know the value of the cosine, sine and tangent of 0, 90 and 180 degrees, as well as the relationships between the lengths of the sides of a right triangle containing angles of 45 or 30 and 60 degrees. This is *essential* for certain physics problems.

7>    Understand the concept of experimental error and be able to calculate it using the appropriate number of significant figures.

8>    Be familiar with vector additions and subtractions. Be able to use the right hand rule. You do not need to know how to calculate the dot or cross product of vectors.

Also:

  *    No knowledge of calculus is required.

  *    Time is a problem for most people taking the MCAT. You should be able to perform the mathematics included in the MCAT quickly. If you have problems with some of the concepts described above, review them. You do not want to have something as elementary as mathematics stop you from doing well.

  *    The math review in this manual is usually presented throughout the science review sections and especially during the Physics and Chemistry reviews. Otherwise, math information can be found in the appendix.

       Please remember the following: if you practice for the MCAT using a calculator then you have not practiced for the MCAT.


<u>Verbal Reasoning</u> (85 minutes)

       This section is designed to measure your ability to read, understand, evaluate and apply information presented in prose texts. The passages are about 500 to 600 words long and are taken from the humanities, social sciences as well as from the natural sciences. Each passage will be followed by six to ten multiple choice questions which will not test you on specific knowledge about a subject. There are a total of 60 questions. All that you need to know to answer the questions will be included in the passage.

### Writing Sample (60 minutes)

Medical schools have noted some deficiencies in the communication skills of their graduates. In response to this problem, an experimental essay writing section was included in the 1991 format of the MCAT. The *new* MCAT includes a writing sample in which you will be asked to write two essays, one in each of two separated half-hour slots. The first essay cannot be returned to you once the second half-hour slot has begun.

The Writing Sample questions consist of a statement which is followed by three writing tasks. The statement will express an opinion, discuss a philosophy or present a policy in a field of general interest. It will not concern an emotionally-charged issue like abortion or religion, or the medical school admission process or your reasons for studying medicine.

The Writing Sample will be scored by two readers who will give your essay a mark from 1 to 6 (best). The mark given will be holistic. If the two marks differ by more than one point, a third reader will be employed to determine the final essay score. The Writing Sample will measure your ability to develop a central idea, to synthesize concepts and to present points clearly and coherently using the accepted rules of grammar, spelling and punctuation.

### Biological Sciences (100 minutes)

The Biological Sciences section is composed of 77 multiple choice questions. There are 62 questions in 10-11 sets of 4 to 8 questions each following a 250-word long passage, and 15 independent questions. The questions concern biology and organic chemistry. Usually, the latter comprises no more than about one quarter to one third of the 77 questions.

As for the Physical Sciences section, some of the questions will assess your ability to read information found in tables, graphs or figures. The biology section of the exam will not test your ability to memorize the name of the 206 bones in the human body or any other highly memory-dependent feat. Rather, it will test your knowledge and understanding of the concepts and principles applicable to the biological sciences, and your problem-solving skills.

Also as in the Physical Sciences section, the questions in the Biological Sciences section cover material learned in elementary level college/university courses. While the passages may present advanced level topics, higher level courses in biology or organic chemistry are not required to take this test. You should know the vocabulary, constants and equations commonly presented in elementary courses. Logic and understanding are emphasized, not memorization. While the amount of material you are responsible for is huge, the actual amount of information you need to know to do well is much more manageable.

## The AAMC

The Association of American Medical Colleges (AAMC) is involved in the development and administration of the *new* MCAT. The AAMC publishes two important sets of materials: i) the *MCAT Practice Items*; and ii) *MCAT Practice Tests* which are released operational test forms from past *new* MCAT administrations. These materials, which also have online test forms, can be obtained by writing or calling:

Membership and Publication Orders
Association of American Medical Colleges
2450 N Street, N.W.
Washington, D.C. 20037-1126
Phone: (202) 828-0416
Web: www.aamc.org

Some students purchase commercially available *simulated* MCAT exams without ever having seen the materials from the AAMC. This is often a serious mistake. If you are looking to write an actual past exam, you go to the source. The source of the MCAT is the AAMC. In this manner, you can feel most confident in your preparedness. The next chapter will provide information regarding *The Gold Standard* which provides explanations to the answers of all the preceding exam materials.

# Chapter 4

# THE RECIPE FOR MCAT SUCCESS

## The Important Ingredients

- Time
- Motivation
- Complete at least 3 of the 4 basic sciences in either university, CEGEP/college, or advanced high-school courses.

- <u>MCAT-Specific Information</u>
  - ‣ The Gold Standard for Medical School Admissions
  - ▷ *optional*: college texts or notes for topics not well understood
  - ▷ *optional*: essay writing or speed reading course if necessary

- <u>MCAT-Specific Problems</u>
  - ‣ The Gold Standard MCAT Practice Exams (GS-1 to GS-6)
  - ‣ The MCAT Student Manual (*available free online at AAMC.org*)
  - ‣ MCAT Practice Items and Practice Tests (*AAMC.org*)
  - ▷ *optional*: online MCAT problems at www.MCAT-prep.com

## The Proper Mix

1)      **Study regularly and start early**.  There is a lot of material to cover and you will need sufficient time to review it all adequately.  Creating a study schedule is often effective.  Starting early will reduce your stress level in the weeks leading up to the exam and may make your studying easier.

2)      **Keep focused and enjoy** the material you are learning.  Forget all past negative learning experiences so you can open your mind to the information with a positive attitude.  Given an open mind and some time to consider what you are learning, you will find most of the information tremendously interesting.  Motivation can be derived from a sincere interest in learning and by keeping in mind your long term goals.

3)      **Biological and Physical Sciences preparation**: *The Gold Standard* is not associated with the AAMC in any way; however, contained within its covers is each and every topic that you are responsible for in the Biological and Physical Sciences, as iterated by the AAMC.  Thus the most directed and efficient study plan is to begin by reviewing the science sections in *The Gold Standard*.

       As you are incorporating the information from the science review, do the Biological and Physical Sciences problems in the Practice Items booklets.  This is the best way to more clearly define the depth of your understanding *and* to get you accustomed to the types of questions you can expect on the MCAT.

**4)**     **Verbal Reasoning and Writing Sample preparation**: Begin by reading the advice given in Chapters 3 and 4 in *The Gold Standard*. Then take the Verbal Reasoning and Writing Sample Practice Items booklet, *always time yourself*, and practice, practice, practice.

For Verbal Reasoning, you should be sure to understand each and every mistake you make as to ensure there will be improvement. For the Writing Sample, you should have someone who has good writing skills read, correct, and comment on your essays. Have the person read Chapter 4 for guidance on what they should be evaluating. And finally, the *MCAT Student Manual*, *Practice Test III* and the latest edition of *The Gold Standard* contain corrected essays which give an indication as to the standard of writing that is expected of you.

**5)**     **Do practice exams**. Ideally, you would finish your science review and Practice Items booklets at least one month prior to the exam date. Then each week you can write 1 or 2 practice exams and thoroughly review each exam after completion. Start with *The Gold Standard* exams GS-1 to GS-4 which will lead you into *Practice Test I* to *V*. The website www.MCAT-prep.com contains GS-5 and 6 as well as essay writing and speed reading courses.

You should write practice exams as you would the actual test: in one sitting within the expected time limits. Writing practice exams will increase your confidence and allow you to see what is expected of you. It will make you realize the constraints imposed by time limits in completing the entire test. It will also allow you to identify the areas in which you may be lacking.

**6)**     **Big on concepts, small on memorization**: Remember that the *new* MCAT will primarily test your understanding of concepts. The *new* MCAT is not designed to measure your ability to memorize tons of scientific facts and trivia, but both your knowledge and understanding of concepts are critical. In fact, only 15% of the science sections on the MCAT <u>directly</u> test your ability to memorize!

Evidently, some material in this manual must be memorized; for example, practically all the science equations, absorption spectra of major functional groups, rules of logarithms, trigonometric functions, the phases in mitosis and meiosis, and other basic facts. Nonetheless, for the most part, your objective should be to try to *understand*, rather than memorize the biology, physics and chemistry material you review. This may appear vague now, but as you write practice material, you will more clearly understand what is expected of you.

**7)**     **Review boo-boos!** Scores in practice exams should improve over time. Success depends on what you do between the first and last exam. Rewriting tests without a systematic review of all mistakes and questionable answers leads to stagnant grades.

**8)**     **Relax once in a while!** While the MCAT requires a lot of preparation, you should not forsake all your other activities to study. Try to keep exercising, maintain a social life and do things you enjoy. If you balance work with things which relax you, you will work more effectively overall.

## It's MCAT Time

1)      On the night before the exam, try to get a good night sleep. The MCAT is physically draining and it is in your best interest to be well rested when you take it.

2)      Avoid last minute cramming. On the morning of the exam, do not begin studying *ad hoc*. You will not learn anything effectively, and noticing something you do not know or will not remember might reduce your confidence and lower your score unnecessarily. Just get up, eat a good breakfast and go write the exam.

3)      Eat breakfast! It will make it possible for you to have the food energy needed to go through the first two parts of the exam.

4)      Pack a light lunch. Avoid greasy food that will make you drowsy. You do not want to feel sleepy for the afternoon sections. Avoid sugar-packed snacks as they will cause a 'sugar low' eventually and will also make you drowsy. A chocolate bar or other sweet highly caloric food could, however, be very useful in the last section (*Biological Sciences*) when you may be tired. The `sugar low' will hit you only after you have completed the exam when you do not *have* to be awake!

5)      Make sure you answer all the questions! You do not get penalized for incorrect answers, so always choose something even if you have to guess. If you run out of time, pick a letter and use it to answer all the remaining questions.

6)      Pace yourself. Do not get bogged down trying to answer a difficult question. If the question is very difficult, make a mark beside it on your exam booklet and answer it later.

7)      Remember that some of the questions will be thrown out as inappropriate or used solely to calibrate the test. If you find that you cannot answer some of the questions, do not despair. It is possible they could be questions used for these purposes.

8)      Do not let others psyche you out! Some people will be saying between exam sections, 'It went great. What a joke!' Ignore them. Often these types may just be trying to boost their own confidence or to make themselves look good in front of their friends. Just focus on what you have to do and tune out the other examinees.

9)      Do not study at lunch. You need the time to recuperate and rest. Eat, avoid the people discussing the test sections and relax!

10)     Before reading the text of the problem, some students find it more efficient to quickly read the questions first. In this way, as soon as you read something in the text which brings to mind a question you have read, you can answer immediately (*this is especially helpful for Verbal Reasoning*). Otherwise, if you read the text first and then the questions, you may end

up wasting time searching through the text for answers. In fact, sometimes in the Physical Sciences and Biological Sciences sections you will be able to answer questions without having read the passage!

11) Read the text and questions carefully! Often students leave out a word or two while reading, which can completely change the sense of the problem. Pay special attention to words in *italics*, CAPS, **bolded,** or underlined. Circle or underline anything you believe might be important in the text or the questions.

12) Do independent questions first! Some students have difficulty finishing the MCAT (esp. Physical Sciences). The worst scenario is getting bogged down in a passage when there were independent questions which you knew the answer to, but never had the time to answer.

13) Expel any *relevant* equation onto your paper! Even if the question is of a theoretical nature, often equations contain the answers and they are much more objective than the reasoning of a nervous pre-medical student! In physics, it is often helpful to draw a picture or diagram. Arrows are valuable in representing vectors.

14) Solving the problem may involve algebraic manipulation of equations and/or numerical calculations. Be sure that you know what all the variables in the equation stand for and that you are using the equation in the appropriate circumstance.

In chemistry and physics, the use of **dimensional analysis** will help you keep track of units and solve some problems where you might have forgotten the relevant equations. Dimensional analysis relies on the manipulation of units. For example, if you are asked for the energy involved in maintaining a 60 watt bulb lit for two minutes you can pull out the appropriate equations or : i) recognize that your objective (unknown = energy) is in joules; ii) recall that a watt is a joule per second; iii) convert minutes into seconds. {note that minutes and seconds cancel leaving joules as an answer}

$$60 \; \frac{joules}{second} \times 2 \; minutes \times 60 \; \frac{seconds}{minute} = 7200 \; joules \; or \; 7.2 \; kilojoules$$

15) The final step in problem solving is to ask yourself: *is my answer reasonable?* For example, if you would have done the preceding problem and your answer was 7200 kilojoules, intuitively this should strike you as an exorbitant amount of energy for an everyday light bulb to remain lit for two minutes! It would then be of value to recheck your calculations. { *'intuition' in science is often learned through the experience of doing many problems*}

16) Whenever doing calculations, the following will increase your speed: (i) manipulate variables but plug in values only when necessary; (ii) avoid decimals, use fractions wherever possible; (iii) square roots or cube roots can be converted to the power (*exponent*) of 1/2 or 1/3, respectively; (iv) before calculating, check to see if the possible answers are sufficiently far apart such that your values can be rounded off (i.e. $19.2 \approx 20$, $185 \approx 200$). In fact, occasionally the MCAT will provide gravity as "given $g = 9.8 \; m/s^2$" but the answers are calculated based on $g = 10 \; m/s^2$!

# Chapter 5

# THE MEDICAL SCHOOL INTERVIEW

*The truth is, that medicine, professedly founded on observation, is as sensitive to outside influences, political, religious, philosophical, imaginative, as is the barometer to the changes of atmospheric density.*

**Oliver Wendell Holmes**, Medical Essays

## Introduction

The application process to most medical schools includes interviews. Only a select number of students from the applicant pool will be given an offer to be interviewed. The medical school interview is, as a rule, something that you *achieve*. In other words, after your school grades, and/or MCAT scores, letters of reference and autobiographical materials have been reviewed, you are offered the ultimate opportunity to put your foot forward: a personalized interview.

Depending on the medical school, you may be interviewed by one, two or several interviewers. You may be the only interviewee or there may be others (i.e., *a group interview*). There may be one or more interviews lasting from 20 minutes to two hours, though 30 minutes is the norm. Despite the variations among the technical aspects of the interview, in terms of substance, most medical schools have similar objectives. These objectives can be arbitrarily categorized into three general assessments: (i) your personality traits, (ii) social skills, and (iii) knowledge of medicine.

**Personality traits** such as maturity, integrity, compassion, sincerity, honesty, originality, curiosity, intellectual capacity, confidence (*not arrogance!*), and motivation are all components of the ideal applicant. These traits will be exposed by the process of the interview, your mannerisms, and the substance of what you choose to discuss when given an ambiguous question. For instance, bringing up *specific* examples of academic achievement related to school and related to self-directed learning would score well in the categories of intellectual capacity and curiosity, respectively.

Motivation is a personality trait which may make the difference between a high and a low or moderate score in an interview. Students must clearly demonstrate that they have the enthusiasm, desire, energy, and interest to survive four long years of medical school and beyond! If you are naturally shy or soft-spoken, you will have to give special attention to this category.

**Social skills** such as leadership, ease of communication, ability to relate to others, volunteer work, cultural and social interests, all constitute skills which are often viewed as critical for future physicians. It is not sufficient to say in an interview: "I have good social skills"! You must display such skills via your interaction with the interviewer(s) and by discussing specific examples of situations which clearly demonstrate your social skills.

**Knowledge of medicine** includes <u>at least</u> a general understanding of what the field of medicine involves, the curriculum you are applying to, and a knowledge of popular medical issues like abortion, euthanasia, AIDS, the health-care system, etc. It is striking to see the number of students who apply to medical school each year whose knowledge of medicine is limited to headlines and popular TV shows! It is not logical for someone to dedicate their lives to a profession they know little about.

Doing volunteer work in a hospital is a good start. This may help clarify your decision for your career choice while providing the admissions committee further evidence of your commitment. Always remember, it is simply not true that a great quantity of volunteer activities secures a position in medical school! As you shall see in the sample interview questions, it is the <u>quality</u> of these experiences which is of greatest value. Alternative ways to enhance your hospital experiences include getting a part-time job in a hospital, or having a relative or family friend who is a physician to help expose you to the daily goings-on in a hospital setting.

Other strategies to keep informed include the following: (i) keep up-to-date with the details of medically related controversies in the news. You should also be able to develop and support opinions of your own; (ii) skim through a medical journal at least once (i.e. the Canadian Medical Association Journal - CMAJ or other medical journal originating from the province where you will be interviewed); (iii) read the medical section of a popular science magazine (i.e. Scientific American, Discover, etc.); (iv) keep abreast of changes in medical school curricula in general and specific to the programs to which you have applied. You can access such information at most university libraries and by writing and/or visiting the web sites of individual medical schools for information on their programs; (v) get some research experience - even if it means volunteering; (vi) do a First-Aid course.

## Preparing for the Interview

If you devote an adequate measure of time for interview preparation, the actual interview will be less tense for you and <u>you</u> will be able to control most of the *content* of the interview.

**Reading** from the various sources mentioned in the preceding sections would be helpful. Also, read over your curriculum vitae and/or any autobiographical materials you may have prepared. Note highlights in your life or specific examples that demonstrate the aforementioned personality traits, social skills or your knowledge of medicine. Zero in on qualities or stories which are either important, memorable, interesting, amusing, informative or "all of the above"! Once in the interview room, you will be given the opportunity to elaborate on the qualities you believe are important about yourself.

**Call the medical school** and ask them about the structure of the interview (i.e., one-on-one, group, etc.) and ask them if they can tell you who will interview you. Many schools have no qualms volunteering such information. Now you can determine the person's expertise by either asking or looking through staff members of the different faculties or medical specialties at that university or college. A cardiac surgeon, a volunteer from the community, and a medical ethicist all have different areas of expertise and will likely orient their interviews differently. Thus you may want to read from a source which will give you a general understanding of their specialty.

**Choose appropriate clothes** for the interview. Every year some students dress for a medical school interview as if they were going out to dance! Medicine is still a conservative profession, you should dress and groom yourself likewise. First impressions are very important. Your objective is to make it as easy as possible for your interviewer(s) to imagine you as a physician.

**Do practice interviews** with people you respect but who can also maintain their objectivity. Let them read this entire chapter on medical school interviews. They must understand that you are to be evaluated *only* on the basis of the interview. On that basis alone, one should be able to imagine the ideal candidate as a future physician.

## Strategies for Answering Questions

Always remember that the interviewer controls the *direction* of the interview by his questions; you control the *content* of the interview through your answers. In other words, once given the opportunity, you should speak about the topics that are important to you; conversely, you should avoid volunteering information which renders you uncomfortable. You can enhance the atmosphere in which the answers are delivered by being polite, sincere, tactful, well-organized, outwardly oriented and maintaining eye contact. Motivation, enthusiasm, and a positive attitude must all be evident.

As a rule, there are no right or wrong answers. However, the way in which you justify your opinions, the topics you choose to discuss, your mannerisms and your composure all play important roles. It is normal to be nervous. It would be to your advantage to channel your nervous energy into a positive quality, like enthusiasm.

**Do not spew forth answers!** Take your time - it is not a contest to see how fast you can answer. Answering with haste can lead to disastrous consequences as happened to a student I interviewed:

Q:    *Have you ever doubted your interest in medicine as a career?*
A:    *No!*
      *Well,...ah...I guess so. Ah ... I guess everyone doubts something at some point or the other...*

Retractions like that are a bad signal but it illustrates an important point: there are usually no right or wrong answers in an interview; however, there are right or wrong ways of answering.  Through the example we can conclude the following: <u>listen carefully to the question</u>, <u>try to relax</u>, and <u>think before you answer</u>!

**Keep on track!**  Unfortunately, some students become so nervous that they entirely forget the question and begin discussing a topic passionately which is completely irrelevant. Keep your mind focused.  Practice should help prevent you from veering off topic and appearing disorganized.

**Do not sit on the fence!** If you avoid giving your opinions on controversial topics, it will be interpreted as indecision which is a negative trait for a prospective physician.  You have a right to your opinions.  However, you must be prepared to defend your point of view in an objective, rational, and informative fashion.  It is also important to show that, despite your opinion, you understand both sides of the argument.  If you have an extreme or unconventional perspective and if you believe your perspective will not interfere with your practice of medicine, <u>you must let your interviewer know that</u>.

For example, imagine a student who was against abortion under *any* circumstance. If asked about her opinion on abortion, she should clearly state her opinion objectively, show she understands the opposing viewpoint, and then use data to reinforce her position.  If she felt that her opinion would not interfere with her objectivity when practicing medicine, she might volunteer: "If I were in a position where my perspective might interfere with an objective management of a patient, I would refer that patient to another physician."

**Carefully note the reactions of the interviewer** in response to your answers. Whether the interviewer is sitting on the edge of her seat wide-eyed or slumping in her chair while yawning, you should take such cues to help you determine when to continue, change the subject, or when to stop talking.  Also, note the more subtle cues.  For example, gauge which topic makes the interviewer frown, give eye contact, take notes, etc.

**Lighten up the interview** with a well-timed story.  A conservative joke, a good analogy, or anecdote may help you relax and make the interviewer sustain his interest.  If it is done correctly, it can turn a routine interview into a memorable and friendly interaction.

It should be noted that because the system is not standardized, a small number of interviewers may ask overly personal questions (i.e., about relationships, religion, etc.) or even questions which carry sexist tones (i.e., *What would you do if you got pregnant while attending medical school?*).  Some questions may be frankly illegal.  If you do not want to answer a question, simply maintain your composure, express your position diplomatically, and address the interviewers <u>real</u> concern (i.e. *Does this person have the potential to be a good doctor?*).  For example, you might say in a non-confrontational tone of voice: "I would rather not answer such a question.  However, I can assure you that whatever my answer may have been, it would in no way affect either my prospective studies in medicine nor any prerequisite objectivity I should have to be a good physician."

## The Group Interview

The great majority of medical school interviews are either one-on-one or two-on-one interviews. Some medical schools, like McMaster's and Laval, have group interviews. Most group interviews consist of 6-8 applicants seated around a table and provided a topic to discuss. The problem may be related to health-care or it may be a 'general interest' story. Members of the admissions committee may either be seated in the room or they may observe the group from behind a two-way mirror. The interviewers are seeing how students interact with their peers, problem solve and how the applicants perform under pressure. Clearly, as for other interviews, one should not show up without reading as much as possible about the philosophy of the school and its current curriculum.

The dynamics of the interview should parallel what is expected from their problem-based learning (PBL) groups. Co-operation leaves no room for loudmouths or people too shy to participate. Your opinion should be presented in a clear, systematic fashion. Keen attention is vital. Only by considering the various opinions can you suggest what the group's opinion is and, in so doing, demonstrate your ability to listen to your peers.

## The Ten Interview Commandments

### Thou shalt not be late.
Yes, every year several students arrive late for one of the most important appointments of their lives. Unquestionably, it is inexcusable. Some medical schools may decide to cancel the application.

### Thou shalt approach and shake the hand.
A confident approach and then a firm, dry (!) handshake leaves a good impression. No Jello handshake nor Arnold Schwartznegger handshake is of any value. Contact has been made.

### Thou shalt pause.
There is no race to answer. Take a few seconds, whether or not you know what you would like to say. Collect your thoughts, gather your composure, then begin.

### Thou shalt maintain eye contact.
Maintaining eye contact achieves two important goals: (1) it demonstrates the confidence you have in what you are speaking about, and (2) it implies sincerity.

### Thou shalt smile.
A smile can allow the interviewer to witness your humanity and watch your ability to 'connect'. A smile may also suggest enthusiasm depending on the nature of the discussion.

### Thou shalt not cry.
Yes, every year some students either begin to tell stories in an interview which they have never told anyone which, because of the elevated activation energy of the interview, occasionally leads to tears. Though it is conceivable that a psychiatrist is conducting the

interview, do not misinterpret the reason that she is there!

## Thou shalt not brag.

I do not believe that students purposefully brag. However, it is quite common for a student to be so uncomfortable about discussing their accomplishments that their manner of speech becomes so awkward that it is often interpreted as arrogance. Ironically, this is precisely what the student was trying to avoid. While it is critical that you describe your accomplishments, it must be done with 'quiet confidence' - without a hint of arrogance. Practice will help you learn to soften the edges. Always remember: what you *learn* from an accomplishment is as important as the accomplishment itself.

## Thou shalt not lie.

In medicine, lives can depend on the truth. If you lie as an applicant, it is in everyone's best interest that you are caught. Here are some classics: (i) students claiming to be able to speak a language other than their mother tongue (i.e. French, Russian, or yes, Swahili) and one of the interviewers happens to speak that language and asks a question which receives no response; (ii) students have claimed to read specific books but when asked about the main characters only a deafening silence answered.

## Thou shalt not assume.

Do not assume that the interviewer, who may be a lay person or a non-science professor, knows acronyms for the names of hospitals, university programs, etc. Also, even if you have submitted autobiographical material, do not assume that they know you. Rather, try to cover a lot of ground about yourself as long as you are concise. The interviewer might relate to something about your history which you did not consider as important. Punctuate your accomplishments with very brief stories which exemplify, without you saying so, traits which are consistent with being a good doctor.

## Thou shalt not be negative.

Some students are consumed with diminishing their accomplishments, self-criticisms, or a string of depressing stories. Thou shalt be positive!

# Chapter 6

# THE INTERVIEW:
# QUESTIONS and ANSWERS

---

*It is our duty to remember at all times and anew that medicine is not only a science, but also the art of letting our own individuality interact with the individuality of the patient.*

Albert Schweitzer

## Sample Questions

There are an infinite number of questions and many different categories of questions. Different medical schools will emphasize different categories of questions. Arbitrarily, ten categories of questions can be defined: ambiguous, medically related, academic, social, stress-type, problem situations, personality oriented, based on autobiographical material, miscellaneous, and ending questions. We will examine each category in terms of sample questions and general comments.

### Ambiguous Questions:

\*\*     *Tell me about yourself.*
         *How do you want me to remember you?*
         *What are your goals?*
         *There are hundreds if not thousands of applicants, why should we*
                 *choose you?*
         *Convince me that you would make a good doctor.*
         *Why do you want to study medicine?*

COMMENTS: These questions present nightmares for the unprepared student who walks into the interview room and is immediately asked: "Tell me about yourself." Where do you start? If you are prepared as previously discussed, you will be able to take control of the interview by highlighting your qualities or objectives in an informative and interesting manner.

### Medically Related Questions:

         *What are the pros and cons to our health-care system?*
         *If you had the power, what changes would you make to our health-care*
                 *system?*
         *Do doctors make too much money?*
         *Is it ethical for doctors to strike?*

*What is the Hippocratic Oath?*
*Should fetal tissue be used to treat disease (i.e. Parkinson's)?*
*If you were a doctor and an under age girl asked you for the Pill (or an abortion) and she did not want to tell her parents, what would you do?*
*Should doctors be allowed to `pull the plug' on terminally ill patients?*
*If a patient is dying from a bleed, would you transfuse blood if you knew they would not approve (i.e. Jehovah Witness)?*

COMMENTS: The health-care system, euthanasia, abortion, human cloning and other ethical issues are very popular topics in this era of technological advances, skyrocketing health-care costs, and ethical uncertainty. You should be up-to-date regarding changes in the province where you are being interviewed. All too often the general public is better informed regarding health-care than the medical school applicant! A well-informed opinion can set you apart from most of the other interviewees.

## Questions Related to Academics:

*Why did you choose your present course of studies?*
*What is your favorite subject in your present course of studies? Why?*
*Would you consider a career in your present course of studies?*
*Can you convince me that you can cope with the workload in medical school?*
*How do you study/prepare for exams?*
*Do you engage in self-directed learning?*

COMMENTS: Medical schools like to see applicants who are well-disciplined, committed to medicine as a career, and who exhibit self-directed learning (i.e. such a level of desire for knowledge that the student may seek to study information independent of any organized infrastructure). Beware of any glitches in your academic record. You may be asked to give reasons for any grades they may deem substandard. On the other hand, you should volunteer any information regarding academic achievement (i.e. prizes, awards, scholarships, particularly high grades in one subject or the other, etc.).

## Questions Related to Social Skills or Interests:

*Give evidence that you relate well with others.*
*Give an example of a leadership role you have assumed.*
*Have you done any volunteer work?*
*What would you do as Prime Minister of Canada with respect to the persistent national debt?*
*How would you address Canada's constitutional crisis?*
*What are the prospects for a lasting peace in South Africa? Eastern Europe? the former USSR? the Middle-East?*
*What do you think of the free-trade agreement between Canada, the United States and Mexico?*

COMMENTS: Questions concerning social skills should be simple for the prepared student. If you are asked a question that you cannot answer, say so. If you pretend to know something about a topic in which you are completely uninformed, you will make a bad situation worse.

**Stress-Type Questions:**

*How do you handle stress?*
*What was the most stressful event in your life? How did you handle it?*
*The night before your final exam, your father has a heart-attack and is admitted to a hospital, what do you do?*

COMMENTS: The ideal physician has positive coping methods to deal with the inevitable stressors of a medical practice. Stress-type questions are a legitimate means of determining if you possess the raw material necessary to cope with medical school and medicine as a career. Some interviewers go one step further. They may decide to introduce stress into the interview and see how you handle it. For example, they may decide to ask you a confrontational question or try to back you into a corner (i.e. *You do not know anything about medicine, do you?*). Alternatively, the interviewer might use silence to introduce stress into the interview. If you have completely and confidently answered a question and silence falls in the room, do not retract previous statements, mutter, or fidget. Simply wait for the next question. If the silence becomes unbearable, you may consider asking an intelligent question (i.e. a specific question regarding their curriculum).

**Questions on Problem Situations:**

*A 68 year-old married woman has a newly discovered cancer. Her life expectancy is 6 months. How would you inform her?*
*A 34 year-old man presents with AIDS and tells you, as his physician, that he does not want to tell his wife. What would you do?*
*You are playing tennis with your best friend and the ball hits your friend in the eye. What do you do?*

COMMENTS: As for the other questions, listen carefully and take your time to consider the best possible response. Keep in mind that the ideal physician is not only knowledgeable, but is also compassionate, empathetic, and is objective enough to understand both sides of a dilemma. Be sure such qualities are clearly demonstrated.

**Personality-Oriented Questions:**

*If you could change one thing about yourself, what would it be?*
*How would your friends describe you?*
*What do you do with your spare time?*
*What is the most important event that has occurred to you in the last*

*five years?*
*If you had three magical wishes, what would they be?*
*What would you do on a perfect day?*
*What are your best attributes?*

COMMENTS: Of course, most questions will assess your personality to one degree or the other. However, these questions are quite direct in their approach. Forewarned is forearmed!

### Questions Based on Autobiographical Materials:

COMMENTS: Any autobiographical materials you may have provided to the medical schools is fair game for questioning. You may be asked to discuss or elaborate on any point the interviewer may feel is interesting or questionable.

### Miscellaneous Questions:

*Should the federal government reinstate the death penalty? Explain.*
*What do you expect to be doing 10 years from now?*
*How would you attract physicians to rural areas?*
*Why do you want to attend our medical school?*
*What other medical schools have you applied to?*
*Have you prepared for this interview?*
*Have you been to other interviews?*

COMMENTS: You will do fine in this grab-bag category as long as you stick to the strategies previously iterated.

### Concluding Questions:

*What would you do if you were not accepted to a medical school?*
*How do you think you did in this interview?*
*Do you have any questions?*

COMMENTS: The only thing more important than a good first impression is a good finish in order to leave a positive lasting impression. They are looking for students who are so committed to medicine that they will not only re-apply to medical school if not accepted, but they would also strive to improve on those aspects of their application which prevented them from being accepted in the first attempt. All these questions should be answered with a quiet confidence. If you are given an opportunity to ask questions, though you should not flaunt your knowledge, you should establish that you are well-informed. For example: "I have read that you have changed your curriculum to a more patient-oriented and self-directed learning approach. I was wondering how the medical students are getting along with these new changes." Be sure, however, not to ask a question unless you are genuinely interested in the answer.

## Answering the Questions

The questions may be seemingly simple. The answers, however, can be a fantastic exercise in clearly demonstrating your commitment to medicine or they could be vague responses drowning in ambiguity. Within seconds of your first response an impression begins to form. At the end of the interview, usually 20 to 45 minutes long, an evaluation will be written that will have a critical impact on your future. For this reason, a couple of points need to be re-emphasized.

There are always two ways that a question is answered in an interview: one is your manner, the other is your words. Consider your manner. Compare one person who speaks in a continuous monotone with few facial expressions while others have multiple inflections when the words leave their lips and begin to smile spontaneously as they describe some aspect of medicine that fascinates them. One student may be viewed as unmotivated while others may seem enthusiastic about medicine.

Manner is also displayed in many other ways including eye contact. Adequate eye contact (not staring!) is often viewed in two important ways for a future doctor: confidence and sincerity. Conversely, shifting one's eyes or looking away from the interviewer while answering a critical question may be seen as unsureness or worse - insincerity. Imagine, all this information that can be derived about your manner alone!

Now let us focus on the content of the answer. Your answer should be clear, to the point and preferably interesting! Begin by listing in your mind the reasons, experiences, anecdotes or analogies that clearly illustrate your interest in medicine. You must be organized and concise. Remember: this is not an interview for McDonald's! The entire medical school interview centers upon one question: *what kind of doctor would you be?*

Some students hold back what they want to say for fear that their answer will sound too sappy! This is supremely ridiculous! If you are being honest, your manner will confirm the sincerity with which you speak.

It is also important to remember that an interviewer will more likely recall a specific example rather than some generalized or ambiguous statement that any student might make.

## Sample Answers: The Good, the Bad and the Ugly

For the proper context it is important to have fully read the two interview chapters. Since there are an infinite number of good, bad and ugly ways to answer a question, do not take the details too seriously. Instead see what you can learn from these specific sample answers which are labelled good (**I**), bad (**II**), or ugly (**III**).

*Tell me about yourself.*          {Interviewer blinded to grades}

**I:**      {pause; total answer less than 4 minutes}
My friends call me Jimmy the Greek.  The odd thing is that I'm not Greek!  They've been calling me that since high-school when we were taught about the Greek scientist Archimedes.  After he had discovered buoyancy for his king, he ran through the streets of Syracuse butt-naked screaming "Eureka, eureka!", which means "I found it".  Certainly my friends do not think of me as the type to run around naked (!), but rather being *enthraled* by what you do - that's who I am.

. . . academic, creative, social . . .

From an academic standpoint, I have always worked hard at school primarily because I love to learn.  I won an entrance scholarship to Simon Fraser University and after a period of adjustment to university life, I was able to give my energies to my craft, and be honored by receiving two more academic awards over the last two years and being placed on the Dean's list.  I am in my last year of an honors program in Life Sciences.

I definitely have a creative side.  I think it's partly due to the years of classical piano lessons.  I learned jazz piano on my own, and I recently had the honour to play with Oscar Peterson at a benefit for cystic fibrosis.  I have also developed creative skills while tutoring, which I thoroughly enjoy, and during research.  I was fortunate to be awarded 2 summer research scholarships during my undergraduate studies to investigate something called *apoptosis*, which is a programmed cell death important in most forms of cancer.  Since this is a relatively new concept, we have had to design new techniques - one of which I had written up and was accepted by the journal Science for publication.  The potential for a treatment for cancer is very exciting.

My social side I express in many ways including with my family, friends and the French and Spanish clubs I've joined at school.  I also play many team sports such as basketball, volleyball and hockey.  My greatest experiences from a social perspective have come from my volunteer activities.  Having volunteered at St. Paul's and the Children's hospital, I have opened a whole new world of possibilities in my personal growth.  I learned to listen to the sick, to hold hands with the elderly, and even to cry with children who saw no hope.  I always did my best to comfort.

It has been said that a doctor may cure sometimes, diagnose often, but comfort always.  I am excited about entering a profession where you can learn, research, teach, and above all, interact in a most human way with those in need.  That is why I am convinced that medicine is the right career choice for me.

**II:**    {no pause}
Dr. Robinson is the main reason I want to be a doctor.  When I was 10 I broke my leg and he was my doctor.  He was really kind and he always had time to listen to my silly complaints.  He went to practice in the States though, but I still remember him as . . .

[Interviewer: "*This is not an interview for Dr. Robinson.  Could you please spend some time talking about yourself?*]

Sorry, it's just that . . . OK . . . I've done a lot of volunteer work, like in the PACU of the VGH and the ER of CHEO, I also have good self-directed learning skills, I'm a good listener, I have leadership skills, I'm good at problem solving, I know these are important to be a good doctor . . . and that's it.

**III:**     {no pause}
Umm, exactly what do you want to know?
            [Interviewer: "*Just tell me about yourself.*"]

Umm, I, I wouldn't know where to start, maybe if you can ask a more specific question.

**Q**: *An eighteen year-old female arrives in the emergency room with a profound nose bleed. You are the physician and you have stopped the bleeding. She is now in a coma from blood loss and will die without a transfusion. A nurse finds a recent signed card from the Jehovah's Witness in the patient's purse refusing blood transfusions under any circumstance. What would you do?*

**I:** {pause}
The courts have recently ruled on this issue saying that a patient has the legal right to refuse treatment, even a life-saving transfusion. As a physician, I would have entered medicine with a purpose - to preserve life. As difficult a decision as it would be for me, I would elect *not* to transfuse. The legal aspect would not influence my decision as much as the *reason* for the law. We live in a multicultural society based on mutual respect. I may not agree with the Sikh who wears a turban into battle, but an adult knows the risks and then balances these with their culture, experiences, and so on. That is their right. I entirely disagree with the idea of refusing a life-saving blood transfusion, all the more painful my decision would be; but on some other day, I will again celebrate the many fascinating differences we have as Canadians.

**II:**     There's no way I would transfuse. She's an adult, it's against the law.

**III:**     I'd give the blood. She's gotta be crazy to believe in that stuff anyways.

# NOTES

# Chapter 7

# AUTOBIOGRAPHICAL MATERIALS

*School yourself to demureness and patience . . .*
*Learn, compare, collect the facts.*

**Ivan Pavlov**, Bequest to the Academic Youth of Soviet Russia

## Introduction

Many medical schools require autobiographical materials as important components of the application process. Autobiographical materials include essays, letters, sketches, or questionnaires where you are given the opportunity to write about yourself. Autobiographical materials are a sort of *written interview*. Thus the same objectives, preparation, and strategies apply as previously mentioned for interviews. However, there are some unique factors.

For example, you can begin writing long in advance of the deadline. The ideal way to prepare is to have a few sheets of paper at home *right now* which you use to continually write any accomplishments or interesting experiences you have had anytime in your life! By starting this process early, months later you should, hopefully(!), have a long list from which to choose information appropriate for the autobiographical materials. Your resume or curriculum vitae may also be of value.

Be sure to write rough drafts and have qualified individuals proofread it for you. Spelling and grammatical errors should not exist.

The document should be written on the appropriate paper and/or in the format as stated in the directions. Do not surpass your word and/or space limit. Ideally, the document would be prepared on a word processor and then laser printed. The document should be so pretty that your parents should want to frame it and hang it in the living room! Handwritten or typed material with 'liquid paper' or 'white-out' is simply not impressive.

## Organization

Your document must be clearly organized. If you are given directive questions then organization should not be a problem. However, if you are given open-ended questions or if you are told, for example, to write a 1000 word essay about yourself, adequate organization is key. There are two general ways you can organize such a response: *chronological* or *thematic*. However, they are not mutually exclusive.

In a chronological response, you are organized by doing a systematic review of important events through time. In writing an essay or letter, one could start with an interesting or amusing story from childhood and then highlight important events chronologically and in concordance with the instructions.

In the **thematic** approach a general theme is presented from the outset and then verified through examples at any time in your life. For example, imagine the following statement somewhere in the introduction of an autobiographical letter/essay:

> *My concept of the good physician is one who has a solid intellectual capacity, extensive social skills, and a creative ability. I have strived to attain and demonstrate such skills.*

Following such an introduction to a thematic response, the essayist can link events from anytime to the general theme of the essay. Each theme would thus be examined in turn.

And finally, keep in mind the advice given for interviews since much of it applies here as well. For example, the appropriate use of an amusing story, anecdote, or an interesting analogy can make your document an interesting one to read. And, as for interviews, specific examples are more memorable than overly generalized statements.

## Sample Successful Autobiographical Materials

*{Note: the following was a 4 page double spaced thematic letter}*

Medicine has been the underlying theme of my life. In fact, as early as kindergarten I would sign my name as "Dr. Nigel" on exams. My teacher interpreted it as my having a sincere interest in medicine (which I did). However, my peers found it to be a bit much in this regard and let me know it in no uncertain manner. As a consequence, I made my first career move: I decided that I would not become a pediatrician! My elder sister recently stated that she had been inspired in part by my early magnetism towards medicine; consequently, she enrolled in a pre-med program at Ottawa University. Dr. Kate Davidson graduated from the University of Toronto in 1990 and went on to McGill to specialize in, of all things, pediatrics!

Since kindergarten I have spent my years cultivating qualities which I feel are important in order to be a successful doctor. Such qualities are: patience and understanding, creativity, leadership and academic achievement.

### Patience and Understanding

I believe that someone who has no predisposition towards patience and understanding could not be a successful medical professional.

In 1990-1991, I worked for five months as a volunteer at the Montreal Association for the Blind. I spent several hours each week with handicapped blind children. Whether one-on-one or in a group, these children thrive on patience and understanding. Regardless of whether I was teaching a child a new chore or a new game, I remember feeling that just one of their smiles was worth all the patience in the world.

To further put such qualities to work, I began tutoring my peers at the Sandy Hill Community Centre (where I function as a Youth Worker and an attendant.) In the last year I have tutored dozens of students in the sciences. I learn as much from them as they do from me. I have learned to develop interpersonal skills such as being able to adapt to the needs of an individual. Most importantly, tutoring taught me, and still teaches me, patience and understanding.

## Creativity

I feel that creativity is an important quality in the study of medicine since it represents the ability to recombine information into new and exciting ways. In this respect I feel that music can serve as a strong analogy.

At the age of twelve, I passed the McGill Conservatory of Music's grade IX examination in classical piano "with honours". With that as a foundation, in 1984 (the Year of the Child), I was offered a fee to compose music and to perform for a theatre group in a summer tour of Canada. Thus, I became a member of Children's Creations.

We performed on the steps of Parliament Hill on Canada Day (introduced by then Prime Minister Turner) and we played as the Tall Ships sailed into Quebec City for Les Voiliers '84. From Place-des-Arts in Montreal to the National Arts Centre in Ottawa; from Klondike Days in Edmonton to the perpetual summer sunlight of Whitehorse; from the metropolis of Toronto to the modesty of Moncton, New Brunswick: we experienced Canada.

While in Toronto, I did interviews for PBS and CBC concerning the tour and its impact on my future. I openly affirmed my desire to enter medicine. I also mentioned that Children's Creations was a beautiful but temporary method to sharpen my creative skills which will one day be used to a greater end.

## Leadership

My last medical examination was sound partly due to my affinity with sports. In high school I was quite athletically successful. I was one of the few individuals who qualified for the Quebec Provincials five years in a row for sports such as basketball, badminton and volleyball.

Due to the size of my high school, many students were not given an opportunity to engage in competitive sports. In order to remedy this, a friend and I set up a "farm system" in which students who were not qualified to splay interscholastically, would play on an intramural team until their skills were sufficiently sharpened. This system is still being employed at my high school where I was also president of the graduating class.

It was more than just new sports organization that I brought to high school, I also brought the publisher of, at the time, the world's second largest francophone publication! Through the help of my English teacher, I organized the play "The Golden Pants" which was written and attended by the publisher of La Presse (Roger Lemelin, author of the play). Mr. Lemelin, after seeing the play, commented on my organizational skills by saying: "You will certainly be the next Prime Minister of Canada!".

Although I was later elected to represent pre-science in the Science Student Association (University of Ottawa), the federal parties have nothing to fear! Since in reality, I was only trying to improve my leadership skills.

**Academic Achievement**

Although I was awarded several academic prizes in elementary and high school, my most valuable achievements came during my university career. Last spring, I was awarded a scholarship from the Association of Professors from the University of Ottawa for the second year in a row. I was chosen for the award based on my first semester GPA of 9.4/10 and an autobiographical letter.

As a result of my average, I was also the recipient of a summer research scholarship from the National Science and Engineering Research Council (NSERC). I spent last summer doing research in the Neurobiology Department of the University of Ottawa. My supervisor, Dr. C. Katinski, was pleased with my work. She was happy that I required little supervision since I feel at home seeking information at the library, doing searches, etc. She has invited me to return next summer with my next NSERC award. She intends to teach me various "patch clamping" techniques which involve some of the most delicate equipment on campus.

I believe academics is important since knowledge is the key to an accurate diagnosis. With this in mind, I decided to broaden my horizons prior to my entry into medical school.

To this end, I will be completing a General B.Sc. with concentration in Life Sciences, though I will be receiving credit for some honours level courses (i.e. neurophysiology). There are fewer than a dozen students registered in my program due to the heavy load of physics and math. However, it is precisely these two subjects which form two of the three integral components of all theories in the fields I hope to study: neurobiology, neurophysiology and neurology. And for the biology component, there will be no lack of it in medical school! Included in my schedule have been several social science disciplines which have been broadening. Presently, I find this little academic experiment to be edifying, enlightening and successful.

Academic achievements come in different forms - some of which never find their way into school transcripts. For example, last fall I received a 90% in the St. John's Ambulance Course. Also, I have written scientific articles in the school's newspaper; some of these articles will be published in the Canadian University Press.

## Conclusion

I have always believed that medicine is the way I could serve society best. Ever since my childhood I have had my eyes focused on medicine. Since then, I have spent much time in many fields, cultivating the qualities I felt were necessary to be the best doctor I could be.

Entering medicine is more than just a childhood dream of mine; rather, it has grown into a lifelong conviction.

*{Note: the following was a 4 page double spaced chronological letter}*

Since my first year of high school in 1988, I knew that I would soon have to make tough career choices. To help me with my decision, I chose a variety of subjects, and participated in many extra-curricular activities. The math and computer science clubs provided opportunities to solve logical problems, while the Reach For The Top team competition tested my knowledge and stimulated my interests in a broad range of topics. The debates set up by the History Department brought out the competitive nature in me, which was also beneficial as a member of the school tennis team. However, this competitive nature was not beneficial in other aspects of my life, especially at the part-time job that I held throughout my high school years.

I started working at a local McDonald's restaurant at age fifteen and by age seventeen, I was a member of the management team. My responsibilities as an assistant manager demanded an ability to communicate and organize. At first, I stumbled, as the competitive nature that I had acquired was becoming noticeable in my work. But gradually, due to experience, and training courses in leadership, I improved. I discovered that working with my fellow employees, and not above or against them, was not only efficient, but also enjoyable. I also began to work more effectively at school, and I started to enjoy team sports such as handball and volleyball.

My interest in science increased throughout my high school years. When it came time to choose a university program, I decided to pursue a B.Sc. In physiology at McGill University. I tried to make my program as variable in content as possible given the restrictions imposed by the program itself. I also decided to participate in a student volunteer program at the Montreal Neurological Hospital with many of the friends that I met in my first year. We talked to several patients each week to try to help relieve some of their loneliness during long hospital stays. The most important thing that I learned from this experience was that, simply listening to and understanding the concern of patients can often make them feel more at ease with their situation. Although, we were able to make some people feel better, I could not help feeling that I wanted to do more. It was at this point that I started to seriously consider medicine as a career.

The many people that I met in my first years to university stimulated a multitude outside interests that I have today. In particular, the appreciation of many forms of music such as folk, reggae, classical and others. Eventually, I learned to play piano and joined a choral ensemble. I also started enjoying many different sports, participating on various intramural teams, cycling regularly, and joining the McGill Tennis Club. Other interests such as snooker, darts and chess can also be attributed to my college experience.

During my second and third years at McGill, I joined a student phone hotline. I received several calls from people trying to adjust to the stress of university life. These conversations further developed my listening and problem-solving skills. I also received calls involving crisis situations, which I feel have helped me react more calmly and constructively when faced with stressful situations.

In my third year at McGill, I was hired as a demonstrator for a first year gross anatomy course. My task was to review with a group of fifteen students, the theory presented in the lectures, while showing them the actual structures inside the human body. The job was easy at first, but as the semester progressed, I had to work several hours each week in order to keep myself one step ahead of my students. Although the work was hard, I discovered that I enjoyed demonstrating immensely and hope to have more chances to teach again in the future.

As I neared the end of my undergraduate work, I still had many tough choices to make. I chose several interesting courses to take in my final year. Many of the courses that I had already taken had given me the opportunity to do many interesting papers and experiments, and I was finding that research could be very creative. Therefore, I considered doing graduate work leading to a Ph.D. in Physiology. I also knew that I had a love for teaching, and so, the idea of becoming a high school teacher was also very appealing. As well, I considered becoming a doctor since I discovered through my volunteer work that helping people could be very rewarding. However, as a result of a personal tragedy, before the start of my final year, I was not prepared to write the MCAT. Since this eliminated my chances of being accepted to McGill's Medical School, I decided to put off applying for one year.

This postponement allowed me the opportunity of taking a closer look at my other career options. After careful consideration, I realized that medicine would allow me to pursue my interests in teaching and research, while at the same time allowing me to utilize and develop the leadership and organization skills that I have been building upon during my school and university years.

I am now convinced that medicine is the right career choice for me, and I have decided against seeking admission to graduate school and Teachers College. Instead, I am spending a year away from school, working full time as a security guard in Toronto. I miss McGill a great deal, and I hope to be back again in September.

# Chapter 8

# LETTERS OF REFERENCE

---

*There is more wisdom in your body than in your deepest philosophy.*

**Friedrich Nietzsche**, Beyond Good and Evil

## Introduction

Letters of reference (a.k.a. *assessments* which are written by *referees*) are required by most medical schools. It provides an opportunity for an admissions committee to see what other people think of you. Consequently, it may be viewed as an important aspect of your application package.

Choose the people who will submit your letter of reference in accordance with instructions from the medical schools to which you are applying. If no such instructions are given, then construct a list of possible referees. Choose from this list individuals who: (i) you can trust; (ii) are reliable; (iii) can write, at least, reasonably well; (iv) understand the importance of your application; and (v) can present with some confidence attributes you have which are consistent with those of a good physician.

Often students either want or are told to have someone as a referee who they do not know well (i.e. a professor). In such a case choose your referee prudently. If they agree to give you a recommendation, give them your resume, curriculum vitae, or any other autobiographical materials you may have. Alternatively, you may ask to arrange a mini-interview. Either way, you would have armed your referee with information which can be used in a specific and personal manner in the letter of reference.

Ideally, one or two of the referees would be professors, and one would be a medical doctor (*either the second professor, a family friend or your own physician*). Clearly, a powerful letter of reference would be one where the author, a doctor, strongly supports the idea of you becoming a doctor. Regarding the professor, if feasible, consider determining if one of your professors is or was a member of the admissions committee. Some professors openly volunteer such information and some medical schools publish the names of the committee members. Once again, such a referee can be very effective.

People are not paid to write you a letter of reference! Therefore, make it as easy as possible for them. Give them an ample amount of time before the deadline for submission. Also, supply them with a stamped envelope with the appropriate address inscribed. Besides being the polite thing to do, they may also be impressed by your organization.  And finally, once the letter of reference has been sent, do not forget to send a "Thank-you" card to your referee.

## Sample Successful Letter of Reference

RE:  Application for Medical School, David Brown

Dr. B. Pritchard
City Hospital
Winnipeg, Manitoba
97/10/10

To whom it may concern,

I have known David and his family for over ten years.  I have watched him grow into a young man who has demonstrated great potential.  He has, over the years, consistently demonstrated a profound interest in science as well as the discipline and tenacity to excel in his studies in order to pursue his dream to study medicine.  His scholastic record and awards speaks to this desire.  However, his academic success is really only an echo of his personal development.  He is a remarkably sincere young man.  His volunteer activities, which I am aware of, have been pursued as a result of a true commitment to community.

It is because of his achievements and my confidence in his self-directed learning skills that he was chosen to be on a team of contributors to The St Paul's Journal (a science review manual).  He spent hundreds of hours during the summer reviewing, synthesizing and even creating some material for the manual.  It is certainly because of his diligence that the material he prepared required relatively minor editing prior to publication.

I am strongly devoted to medicine and can sense when others share this passion.

David has shown a great degree of maturity and passion for medicine.  As a result of my familiarity with David, I can say with confidence, were he a physician, it would be my honor for him to be my physician.


Ben Pritchard BSc MD ('67)

**THE BLACK BOOK**

# Chapter 9

# THE INTERNET

---

*In teaching the medical student the primary requisite is to keep him awake.*

**Chevalier Jackson**, The Life of Chevalier Jackson

## Welcome to the Information Age . . .

The internet has revolutionized many aspects of industry. It is a growing force in medicine as doctors from around the world can video conference essentially for free, log on to clinical problems presented with X-rays, CAT scans and MRIs from other hospitals, and gain access to the latest abstracts from almost any medical journal in an instant. Teaching medicine will certainly change in part because of this powerful tool.

On the other hand, the same warnings must be kept in mind as for any other industry: beware of the *source* of information. As you read through the book you will find internet addresses which you should really spend some time exploring. These include the web sites of many Canadian medical schools, OMSAS (**http://www.ouac.on.ca**), AAMC (**http://www.aamc.org**), etc. Certainly these are dependable sources. The following are some interesting internet addresses of varying degrees of utility and dependability. Almost all the sites are 'free'.

I have been involved in designing: **http://www.futuredoctor.net**. This free site contains access routes to the ratings of American medical schools (US News & World Report), AMCAS, the New England Journal of Medicine, advice for autobiographical materials, medical school web sites and much more. Some of the medical school web sites are excellent. Writing Sample advice can be accessed at **WritingSample.com**. When you are going for your medical school interviews log on and get access to the latest interview questions from Canadian and American medical schools at **http://www.studentdoctor.net/**. The latter can be found through many premed search engines.

You can get tips for interviews and autobiographical essays at another US internet site: **http://premed.com/docs/advisor.html**. General application advice, but especially essays, can be found at: **http://premed.edu/essay.html**. Upon review, the whole **http://premed.edu/** site is quite innovative and informative.

A fairly good Canadian site generated by a medical student at UBC can be found at: **http://www.geocities.com/hotsprings/oasis/8998/frames.html**.

Free MCAT exams can be downloaded from the internet by putting the keyword "MCAT" in your search engine. The exams are currently free from the AAMC (one real past

MCAT), Kaplan and Princeton Review. However, beware of exams which are constructed to have you conclude that you should take their course. Remember: actual past MCATs always supercede simulations. Some brief MCAT science review information can be downloaded from: **http://www.cris.com/~Ourmazdi/biology/biology.htm**, currently a free internet site.

If you go to the OMSAS website previously mentioned, there is a link to Queen's medical school which provides the best explanation of problem-based learning available online.

If I ever come to your town to give lectures regarding medical school admissions or the MCAT, you will be the first to know at **http://www.prep.com**. There you will find links to Canadian premed websites which you may find helpful. The **http://www.MCAT-prep.com** site will give you access to online MCAT lectures. If you have any comments about the book or other interesting experiences or web sites you would like to share, drop a line at the following e-mail address: **ruveneco@bellnet.ca**.

# Chapter 10

# THE EVOLUTION OF THE CANADIAN MEDICAL SCHOOL

---

*The successful teacher is no longer on a height, pumping knowledge at high pressure into passive receptacles . . . He is a senior student anxious to help his juniors.*

**Sir William Osler** (1849-1919), Internationally-acclaimed Canadian physician

## In the Beginning . . .

At the turn of the nineteenth century, becoming a physician in Canada was relatively simple: either you came from a wealthy family or you encountered a doctor who was impressed by you. Given that there were no universities in Canada at the time, no undergraduate degree was necessary! Medical education involved a few years as an apprentice with an established medical practitioner. After which, 'the graduate' may decide to pursue further studies abroad or simply begin a medical practice. A significant number of 'doctors' at the time were charlatans with no training whatsoever.

In Montreal between 1818 and 1822, several physicians laid the groundwork to standardize the evaluation of applicants to practice medicine and to create Canada's first medical school. Thus in 1822 the Montreal General Hospital, equipped with a Board of Medical Examiners, opened its doors. By execution of the will of James McGill in 1829, land was provided for the opening of McGill University whose original faculty was that of the Faculty of Medicine.

The sixty years which followed resulted in the emergence of seven Canadian medical schools from Nova Scotia to Manitoba: University of Montreal (francophone) and University of Toronto in 1843, University of Laval (francophone) in 1852, Queen's University in 1854, Dalhousie University in 1868, University of Western Ontario in 1882, and the University of Manitoba in 1883.

## The Flexner Report

Abraham Flexner was a professional educator who was hired by the Carnegie Foundation for the Advancement of Education to evaluate the condition of medical education in America and to make suggestions for the future. His report was published in 1910 and would stand as the gold standard on medical education for decades.

For his evaluation Flexner visited the medical schools in both Canada and the US. He was not known for mincing his words. Regarding one medical school, he wrote:

*"Entrance requirement: Less than a high school education."*

And yet another:

*"The school occupies a few neglected rooms on the second floor of a fifty-foot frame building. Its so-called equipment is dirty and disorderly beyond description. Its outfit in anatomy consists of a small box of bones and the dried-up fragments of a single cadaver. A few bottles of reagents constitute the chemical laboratory. A cold and rusty incubator, a single microscope, and a few unlabelled wet specimens, etc., form the so-called 'equipment' for pathology and bacteriology."*

## Borderline to Excellence

In order to prepare his report, Flexner visited all eight Canadian medical schools in 1909. He regarded the programs at McGill and Toronto as first class. He thought Queen's and Manitoba had given a good effort but had fallen short. In fact, because of unstable funding and a small clinical base, he felt there was no future for a medical school at Queen's. Flexner deemed Western and Dalhousie "feeble proprietary schools." He felt Canada's two francophone medical schools, Laval and Montreal, should merge since neither stood well on its own. Many feel that his criticisms served as a catalyst for change and improvement. Flexner could not have foreseen how all eight medical schools would make their mark on the world stage.

In his report, Flexner's most scathing comments were directed towards American medical schools. He concluded that there were too many medical schools, many were substandard, and prerequisites for the study of medicine and the content of medical education had to be defined. He suggested that the minimum requirement for admissions to medical school include a high school diploma and two years of a college or university level science curriculum.

He recommended that medical school be four years long. The first two years would involve the basic sciences with relevant laboratories. The first year would include anatomy, histology, embryology, physiology and biochemistry. The second year would explore pathology, bacteriology, pharmacology and physical diagnosis. The last two years would be clinical. Thus in the last two years learning would occur through experience garnered on hospital wards and dispensaries. Flexner's 'two plus two' solution to medical education formed the bedrock for teaching medicine in Canada for decades.

Within 20 years of the Flexner Report, unlike in the US, all eight Canadian medical schools not only survived, but each received Class A status according to the American Medical Association. Rather than losing any medical schools, the University of Alberta opened its doors to medical education in 1913.

After decades of following Flexner's recommendations remarkably close, only relatively recently have Canadian medical schools turned away from the Flexner Report, probing, exploring, and creating new paths towards medical education.

## The Canadian Spirit of Innovation

In 1951, the Massey Commission recommended federal support for Canadian universities. This led to a period of expansion during the 1950s and 1960s for the established medical schools. These boom years also led to the birth and/or growth of the University of Ottawa (1945), the University of British Columbia (1950), and the University of Saskatchewan (1953).

In 1964, the Hall Commission recommended the introduction of universal health-care which the government approved. The Commission also made projections based on population shifts, demographics and physician access. In its conclusions, the Commission recommended that a historic $500 million Health Resources Fund be created to fund new medical buildings, new teaching hospitals and even new medical schools. Thus resources were made available for the inauguration of Canada's 'new medical schools': University of Sherbrooke (1966), Memorial University (1969), McMaster University (1969) and University of Calgary (1970). The latter having broken away from the University of Alberta (founded in 1913).

On the political side, years of pioneering work led to North America's first government-administered medical insurance plan in Saskatchewan in 1962. As the backdrop to the development of the new medical schools, one finds newly elected Prime Minister Pierre Trudeau. In 1968, after years of seemingly stalled legislation, Trudeau signed Canada's Health-Care Act into law providing all our citizens with first-class health-care. Medicare was born as a national entity and the experiment in the universality of health-care began. Canadian innovation would continue, but now at the level of the medical schools .

The new schools had no problem attracting staff, from the older medical schools, interested in change. Flexner's outline of medical education would be forever altered in Canada by those willing to consider and enact an alternative form of education. Two of the four new schools generated *three* year programs based on 11 months of education per year (McMaster and Calgary). All four medical schools graduated their first class between 1970 and 1973, taught the sciences based on body systems, and used problem-based learning. These latter concepts are also used in Canada's newest medical school (2004): the Northern Ontario Medical School (NOMS) based in Sudbury and Thunder Bay. The latter finally addresses the deficit many northern communities have in terms of access.

## The New Schools

The new medical schools based their curricula on body systems. The classic education at the time followed Flexner's prescription, as previously described, thus courses were parallel but independent. This meant that in the same time period, *each* professor would attempt to present the exponential growth of material with little or no restriction. This resulted, on the whole, with the teaching of information during Flexner's basic science years which was, at best, only slightly relevant to both medical practice and licensing exams.

The body systems approach integrated the various disciplines into an organized framework. For example, a period of time could be set aside to learn about the cardiovascular system. Thus the system would be viewed from the perspective of the various disciplines - anatomy, physiology, etc. This teaching method is more efficient, less repetitive. Decisions must be made regarding the quantity and quality of the information being taught and its relevance to a future practitioner. Some of the older schools, including Dalhousie, Laval, Montreal, Ottawa, and Toronto, began adopting a similar integrated approach.

The new schools all used a problem-based approach to education. McMaster University is most well known for its development and for advising other medical schools (i.e. Harvard) on how to set up a similar system. The problem-based learning (PBL) approach relies on people. The cornerstone is no longer the building, the faculty nor the equipment. The basis for the education is the student, the rest is the supporting cast. As the antithesis to the lecture hall, students are assembled into small groups of 6-8 students and are presented with real clinical scenarios. The challenge is to solve the problem with no medical experience. This requires team-work in order to cooperate and divide labor; self-directed learning to access and understand the information (a skill which is vital for the practicing physician); and finally, back to the team to teach, to learn, and to consolidate.

Neame *et al* iterated the following questions which a group of students involved in problem-based learning might be expected to address, with regard to a specific clinical problem:

- What might have caused the complaint?
- What is the best way to differentiate between the possible causes?
- What is the pathophysiological mechanism responsible for the complaint and clinical condition?
- How might it best be managed?
- What brought it on, and how?
- How might it be prevented from occurring/recurring and/or earlier detected for treatment?

Thus the changes in medical education, in large part secondary to the new schools, have been quite significant. The body systems approach, problem-based learning, and other innovations like the early immersion of medical students into hospitals and other clinical settings (*another anti-Flexner development*) have been slowly spreading throughout

Canadian medical schools. Never has metastasis been so welcome.


## The Future of Canadian Medical Schools

Undoubtedly, the future is bright, exciting and full of challenges. The brief historical outline in this chapter has not the breadth to illustrate the very dark times in the histories of most Canadian medical schools. There were instances when the future was counted in weeks not decades or centuries. And yet the record displays growth, achievement, world-wide recognition, and most importantly, consistent and excellent provision of health-care to our communities. All Canadian medical schools have a Class A rating and all are regarded as "Strong" by the Gourman Report, which gives all Canadian medical schools higher ratings than the majority of US medical schools.

The challenges, however, are significant. History suggests that the challenges shall be met, handily. The following includes a few of the many issues which Canadian medical schools are summoned to face:

- The changing medical school curriculum: new ideas vs. proponents of inertia
- Specialization and new residency programs
- The research explosion: potential and expansion vs. fiscal responsibility and cutbacks
- The unresolved issue of the ideal physician/population ratio
- Positions cut in the cities, insufficient staff in rural areas
- Fewer applicants and fewer positions in medical schools
- Getting the government and the public interested in preventative medicine
- Hospital closures
- Complex ethical issues
- Maintenance of Medicare
- Doctors' salaries
- Alternative medicine: hoax vs. coverage under Medicare


## Provincial Barriers

Education and health are the domain of the provinces. Medical schools are expensive, as are doctors. In this era of deficit reduction, provincial health-care ministers continually re-evaluate the number of positions in medical schools, funding, doctors' salaries, etc. 'Cost-cutting' has led to reductions in positions at medical schools across the country.

Certainly, therefore, out-of-province students can quickly become expendable as a result of decisions made by short-sighted politicians. A classic example is that of a letter written by Ontario's former Health-care Minister Ruth Grier to her Quebec counterpart Marc-Yvan Côté, asking Quebec to diminish the numbers of Ontario students at Quebec medical schools. The situation escalated to a complete ban on out-of-province students being admitted to Quebec schools. Only in politics could the following be rationalized: in 1995 no Canadian residents from outside Quebec were permitted to attend Quebec medical schools; however, up to 30 citizens of other countries were permitted to attend medical schools in Montreal, Sherbrooke, or Quebec City. C'est la vie.

Quebec has re-opened its doors, somewhat. British Colombia has been the stingiest. Clearly the issue remains unresolved: what are the responsibilities of a medical school to its community and to all Canadians, including prospective medical students? In all likelihood the answer will be provided by the government, not the medical schools. As regrettable as it has been, fortunately the provincial barriers have been for students, not ideas.

# The MSPC
# DIRECTORY:
# *MEDICAL SCHOOLS in*
# *NORTH AMERICA*

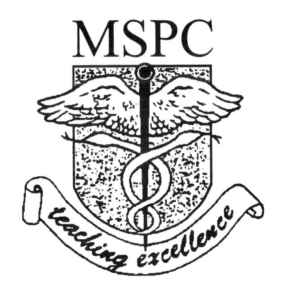

# Chapter 11

# THE CANADIAN MEDICAL SCHOOLS

---

*Tie off pancreas ducts of dogs.  Wait six to eight weeks.  Remove and extract.*

**Frederick G. Banting,** Canadian surgeon who discovered insulin, Nobel Prize for Medicine in 1923

## From East to West

- Memorial University
- Dalhousie University
- Université Laval
- Université de Sherbrooke
- Université de Montréal
- McGill University
- University of Ottawa
- Queen's University
- University of Toronto
- McMaster University
- University of Western Ontario
- Northern Ontario Medical School
- University of Manitoba
- University of Saskatchewan
- University of Alberta
- University of Calgary
- University of British Colombia

# NOTES

# Memorial University of Newfoundland

- ## Address for Inquiries and Applications
  Admissions Office
  Memorial University of Newfoundland
  Faculty of Medicine,
  Health Sciences Center, Room 2701
  St. John's, Newfoundland, Canada A1B 3V6
  (709) 777-6615; 777-6396 (FAX)
  E-mail: munmed@mun.ca
  Web site: http://www.med.mun.ca

- ## Application Deadline
  October 15th

- ## Required to Submit
  Application form and fee
  1 copy of post secondary academic transcript
  2 letters of reference
  MCAT score must be reported by mid-December prior to anticipated entrance.
  Interview may be requested.

- ## Academic Requirements
  A bachelor degree and the MCAT are required. Special circumstances exist, however, enabling certain students to be considered who have completed only 20 one-semester courses, which is 2 full years of university work. In both cases a minimum of two English courses are required. The preceding prerequisite is equivalent to English in 2 semesters of undergraduate studies or one year of OAC grade XIII (Ontario) or 4 courses in CEGEP (Quebec).

- ## Required Academic Standing (GPA)
  An overall average of 80% is common (or equivalent in other grading systems). Usually out-of-province students require 83 - 85%.

- ## Average MCAT Score
  The average MCAT score is 9 on each section (2004). Students with an MCAT score of 8 or better on each section and a letter grade of "O" in the Writing Sample are considered "academically competitive" in the selection process.

- ## Number of Students Accepted to Faculty
  60

- **Length of Program**
  4 years

- **Application Fee**
  $75

- **Tuition Fee**
  Canadian students: $6,250
  International students: $30,000

- **Can acceptance be deferred?**
  Requests are considered.

- **Province of Residence**
  Usually 40 seats are given to residents of Newfoundland, Labrador, NB (10), and PEI (2); 15 seats go to foreign students and 5 to out-of-province applicants.
  These figures may change from year to year.

## What you should know about Memorial University

- The Gourman Report ranks the medical school at Memorial University of Newfoundland in the category "Strong"; score: 4.37/5.0.
- During the selection process, the admissions committee places considerable weight on MCAT scores, academic achievement as well as on one's academic background of study (degree of difficulty and course load are important). Letters of reference and in some case interviews are used to determine a candidate's personal characteristics, motivation, and personal achievements.
- Re-applications are accepted the next academic year without prejudice.
- Sex, age, race, religion nor marital status are considered in the selection process.
- Combined MSc or PhD programs are available.
- Every course taken since high school is considered and reviewed by the committee.

# Dalhousie University

- ## Address for Inquiries and Applications
  Brenda L. Detienne, Admissions Coordinator
  Room C-132 Lower level, Clinical Research Center
  5849 University Avenue, Dalhousie University, Halifax
  Nova Scotia, Canada, B3H 4H7
  (902) 494-2450; 494-6369 (FAX)
  E-mail: brenda.detienne@dal.ca
  Web site: http://www.medicine.dal.ca

- ## Application Deadline
  October 31st

- ## Required to Submit
  Application form and fees
  3 confidential assessments to be sent directly to the University
  MCAT scores
  1 official copy of grades from all universities and colleges attended
  If a student is still in the process of attending university, an interim transcript is to be sent with application, and a final official transcript is to be sent upon completion of studies.
  Autobiographical essay and sketch (activity profile)
  Interviews (selected applicants)

- ## Academic Requirements
  Minimum requirement is a completed undergraduate bachelor's degree (with no specific prerequisites; 4 year degree is preferable), and the writing of the MCAT within the last 5 years.

- ## Required Academic Standing (GPA)
  In each of the last 2 consecutive full-time years:
  - Maritime applicants must have a minimum of B+ (77% or GPA of 3.30).
  - Non-Maritime applicants must have a minimum of A- (80% or GPA of 3.70).

- ## Average MCAT Score
  Maritime applicants must have a minimum of 8 in any 2 sections (min. total = 24 for the three multiple-choice sections).
  Non-Maritime applicants must have a min. of 10 in any 2 sections (min. total = 30).

- ## Number of Students Accepted to Faculty
  90

- **Length of Program**
  4 years

- **Application Fees**
  $65

- **Tuition Fees**
  Canadian students: $8,800
  International students: $30,000

- **Can acceptance be deferred?**
  Acceptance may be deferred for one year in unusual circumstances.

- **Province of Residence**
  Preference is given to Canadian citizens or landed immigrants who reside in Nova Scotia, New Brunswick or Prince Edward Island. Seventy-four places are reserved for the residents of these maritime provinces. Up to 10% of entering places will be considered for qualified, out-of-province candidates.

## What you should know about Dalhousie University

- The Gourman Report ranks the medical school at Dalhousie University in the category "Strong"; score: 4.33/5.0.
- There are no pre-requisites other than a baccalaureate degree for entrance into Dalhousie's Faculty of Medicine. The MCAT is an absolute requirement.
- Courses taken in humanities and social sciences are looked upon as helpful toward understanding human behaviour.
- Excellent communication skills are expected verbally as well as written.
- A good record of achievement in academic as well as non-academic activities is sought.
- No discrimination is made on the basis of sex, race, creed, are, national origin or handicap.
- More emphasis is put on the last 2 years of academic study. A transcript with failed classes, repeated courses, supplementary exams, or low grades within the last two years of study, greatly diminish the candidates chance of admission.
- Individual merits are considered from applicants of minority groups once they have met the minimum requirements.
- For those who wish to re-apply, a new form must be re-submitted each year.
- Students with learning disabilities may apply under "special circumstances."
- Successful applicants are expected to send a $200 deposit to ensure their place at the university, this fee is later applied to tuition.
- Case-Oriented Problem Stimulated Learning (COPS; cf. PBL) is now integrated into the curriculum.

# Université Laval

- ## Address for admissions
  Bureau du régistraire
  Pavillon Jean-Charles-Bonenfant
  Université Laval
  Quebec, Canada, G1K 7P4
  (418) 656-3080
  Courrier électronique: fmed@fmed.ulaval.ca
  Web site: http://www.fmed.ulaval.ca

- ## Address for Inquiries
  Secretaire du Comité d'admission
  Faculté de médecine
  Pavillon Vandry
  Université Laval
  Quebec, QC, G1K 7P4
  (418) 656-2131 (2492)

- ## Application Deadline
  Quebec residents: March 1st
  International and out-of-province Canadian students: January 1st

- ## Required to Submit
  Application form and fee
  1 copy of post-secondary academic transcript
  A standardized C.V.
  2 letters of reference
  1 personal statement
  ABS Test (Assessment by Stimulation): a three-hour group session conducted to evaluate various behavioral characteristics of applicants.

- ## Academic Requirements
  Fluency in French is mandatory.
  2 full years of College (i.e. CEGEP) in the Faculty of Health Sciences resulting in a diploma (DEC), or a university degree, or 75 credits at the time of submission of the application is acceptable. The equivalent from other schools outside of Quebec are determined to be acceptable or not by the registrars office of the university. The following courses are compulsory:
  - Two Biology courses (with lab): BIO 301 and BIO 401
  - Two Math courses: MAT 103 and MAT 203
  - Three Chemistry courses (with lab): CHM 101, CHM 201 and CHM 202
  - Three Physics courses (with lab): PHY 101, PHY 201 and PHY 301

- **Required Academic Standing (GPA)**
  N/A

- **Average MCAT Score**
  N/A
  The MCAT is not required; however, it is taken into consideration if submitted with the application.

- **Number of Students Accepted to Faculty**
  189

- **Length of Program**
  4 years

- **Application Fee**
  $30

- **Tuition Fees**
  Canadian student tuition fees are approximately $3,248
  International student fees are approximately $15,000.

- **Can acceptance be deferred?**
  No deferrals are permitted.

- **Province of Residence**
  144 seats are reserved for Quebecois students and 5 seats are allocated to applicants from New Brunswick (2001).

- **Formula for Admissions**
  The first cutoff is based on academic ability as reflected in the 'côte de rendement'. The latter is based on academic transcripts and a statistical comparison of performance. The top 315 applicants receive further evaluation.
  The formula for university degree holders is as follows: 50% is based on academic ability, the ABS test result accounts for 25%, and the remaining 25% is based on the candidate's C.V.
  CEGEP and university students are similarly evaluated but instead the ABS test result accounts for 30%, and 10% is based on the candidate's standardized personal statement.

### What you should know about the Université Laval

- The Gourman Report ranks the medical school at the University of Laval in the category "Very Strong"; score: 4.62/5.0.
- All instruction at the university is in French. All successful applicants must take the "Test de Ministère de l'Enseignement supérieur et de la science," to prove competency

in French. Knowledge of the English language is recommended.
- Sex, race, religion, socioeconomic status and age are not criteria in the selection process.
- The university aims at integrating handicap students who wish to study medicine yet who's disability does not interfere with the practice.
- The university usually provides 63% of positions to CEGEP graduates and 37% of positions to those with a bachelor's degree from university.
- A combined MD/PhD program is available.

# NOTES

# Université de Sherbrooke

- ## Address for Inquiries and Applications
  Admissions Office, University of Sherbrooke
  Faculty of Medicine, Sherbrooke, Quebec
  Canada J1H 5N4; (819) 564-5208; 564-5378 (FAX)
  E-mail: admmed@courrier.usherb.ca
  Web site: http://www.usherb.ca

- ## Application Deadline
  March 1st

- ## Required to Submit
  Application form and fee
  1 birth certificate
  1 copy of all post-secondary transcripts
  an aptitude test

- ## Academic Requirements
  Two years of college is the minimum requirement (CEGEP). Those entering with a diploma (DEC) must have majored in sciences and completed 'bloc 10.11'. A diverse background should be demonstrated in the Humanities such as: literature and philosophy. Expected in the behavioural and social sciences are courses such as: sociology, history and psychology.
  Those with a B.A. or a B.Sc. are required to have done 2 semesters of each of the following:
  General Biology (lab incl.)
  General Chemistry (lab incl.)
  Organic Chemistry (lab incl.)
  And 3 semesters of each of the following:
  General Physics (lab incl.) and
  Mathematics through calculus (college algebra, analytical geometry and trigonometry).

- ## Required Academic Standing (GPA)
  Selection procedures are presently being revised.

- ## Average MCAT Score
  The MCAT is not required.

- ## Number of Students Accepted to Faculty
  130

- ## Length of Program
  4 years

- ## Application Fees
  $30

- ## Tuition Fees
  Canadian students: $3 019.38
  International students: $15 019.38

- ## Can acceptance be deferred?
  No

- ## Province of Residence
  18 out of province students were accepted in 2001.

- ## Formula for Admissions
  75% GPA + 25% aptitude test

## What you should know about the University of Sherbrooke

- The Gourman Report ranks the medical school at the University of Sherbrooke in the category "Strong"; score: 4.25/5.0.
- All applicants must be proficient in the French language. Any accepted applicant who has completed previous studies in a language other than French is required to take a test to assess their competency in French, an 84% must be attained in order to be accepted to the University.
- Admission is primarily based on academic achievement, however, the selection process is currently being reviewed and revised due to the new curriculum of medical studies. Presently, applicants who are applying directly from CEGEP are primarily assessed on the scholastic record they submit.
- For those applicants who have attended university the criteria is as follows: 0% = CEGEP transcript and 100% = undergraduate GPA.
- No transfers are accepted.
- A learning skills test will now be part of the application procedure.
- A combined MD/MSc program is available.

# Université de Montréal

- ## Address for Inquiries
  University of Montreal
  Faculty of Medicine, C.P. 6128, Succursale A
  Montreal, Quebec, Canada H3C 3J1
  (514) 343-6265/7076; 343-6629 (FAX)
  E-mail: admmed@ere.umontreal.ca
  Website: www.umontreal.ca

- ## Address for Applications
  Services des admissions
  Bureau du régistraire
  Université de Montreal
  C.P. 6205, Succursale A
  Montreal, QC, H3C 3T5

- ## Application Deadline
  March 1st

- ## Required to Submit
  Application form and fee
  1 copy of post-secondary school transcripts
  Interview

- ## Academic Requirements
  Pre-requisites are: fluency in the French language, a minimum of 2 years of study at the college level (CEGEP) in Health Sciences and a DEC (collegial studies of the Department of Education). Courses taken should include philosophy, French, English, behavioral and social sciences, mathematics (trigonometry, calculus, college algebra and analytical geometry) and sciences (biology, inorganic and organic chemistry and physics).

  A preparatory year (*premed*) is mandatory at this university, the only students who may directly enter the 4 year MD program are those with one of the credentials listed below:

  baccalauréat en biochimie

  baccalauréat en ergothérapie

  baccalauréat en nutrition

  baccalauréat en orthophonie-audiologie

  baccalauréat en pharmacie

  baccalauréat en sciences biologiques

  baccalauréat en science infirmières

  doctorat en médecine dentaire

  doctorat en optométrie

  doctorat en médecine vétérinaire

  baccalauréat en physiothérapie

- **Required Academic Standing (GPA)**
  N/A

- **Average MCAT Score**
  The MCAT is not required.

- **Number of Students Accepted to Faculty**
  227

- **Length of Program**
  4 years (5 years if pre-medical courses are needed; *see* Academic Requirements).

- **Application Fees**
  $30

- **Tuition Fees**
  Canadian residents: $2,480
  International students: $13,812

- **Can acceptance be deferred?**
  No

- **Province of Residence**
  Canadian citizens or landed immigrants are given priority, however, consideration is also given to French speaking applicants from other provinces and from the US as well.

- **Formula for Admissions**
  For applicants applying directly from CEGEP or university the selection criteria is the same: (1) approximately one quarter of the applicants with the highest grades will be invited for an interview; (2) the final global score for admissions: 50% = academic achievement and 50% = the interview.
  University applicants who have completed a PhD or whose thesis will be submitted prior to admission, have their global score based 50% on their research work and 50% on the interview.

## What you should know about the University of Montreal

- The Gourman Report ranks the medical school at the University of Montreal in the category "Very Strong"; score: 4.78/5.0.
- Proficiency in the French language is required, all successful candidates who have not studied in French in the last two years prior to applying must take a test administered by the university to prove their competence in French.

- Selection is primarily based upon academic achievement and on an interview.
- Race, sex, creed or age are not considered in the selection process.
- Three seats are offered to francophone residents of New Brunswick, and one seat is offered to a qualified francophone resident of Prince Edward Island (most likely the three seats reserved for residents of N.B. will no longer be available for 1998/99 and beyond). However, extra seats will be made available at the University of Sherbrooke.
- Four seats are often offered to foreign students with a visa.
- Combined MD/MSc and MD/PhD programs are available.
- In 2001-2002, 189 students were accepted to first year courses.
- Transfers are a possibility.

# McGill University

- ## Address for Inquiries and Applications

  Admissions Office, McGill University
  Faculty of Medicine, 3655 Drummond Street
  Montreal, Quebec, Canada  H3G 1Y6
  (514) 398-3515; 398-4631 (FAX)
  E-mail: medadm@medcor.mcgill.ca
  Website: www.med.mcgill.ca

- ## Application Deadline

  January 15th for residents of Quebec applying for the 4 year program;
  March 1st for those applying to the 5 year program;
  November 15th for applicants to the MD/MBA program,
  the MD/PhD program, and for all applicants from outside of Quebec

- ## Required to Submit

  Application form and fees
  1 copy of post-secondary academic transcript(s)
  1 autobiographical letter
  3 letters of reference
  MCAT score report (university applicants only)
  Interviews are conducted.

- ## Academic Requirements

### FOUR YEAR PROGRAM

At the time of application an undergraduate degree with full course load must be in the final year of completion, or should be completed.

Applicants from the province of Quebec must have completed 90 credits (equivalent to six semesters, three years) in a Quebec university.

Applicants from outside the province of Quebec must have completed 120 credits (equivalent to eight semesters, four years) in a university.

Specific requirements are one full university year with laboratory work in: general biology, general chemistry, organic chemistry and physics.

Strongly recommended: a university level semester in: cell biology and molecular biology (a full year course in biochemistry can be substituted for the latter two mentioned).

### FIVE YEAR PROGRAM

Citizens or permanent residents of Quebec residing in the province who are completing their final year of "Sciences de la Nature" from select CEGEP's can apply to this five year program.

Required courses - Bloc 10.11
Biology 301, 401
Chemistry 101, 201, 202
Mathematics 103, 203
Physics 101, 201, 301
Chemistry 302 is recommended

## • Required Academic Standing (GPA)

**FOUR YEAR PROGRAM**
Candidates are expected to have a GPA of 3.5 or better on a 4.0 scale. The first year classes of 1996-97 to 2000-01 had an average of approximately 3.7/4.0. The 2002-2003 mean CGPA was 3.80.

**FIVE YEAR PROGRAM**
A minimum overall average of 85% is required.

## • Average MCAT Scores

A combined score of 30 or more in the three multiple choice sections of the MCAT is expected.
Mean scores of the entering class of 2001-02 (2002-03 in brackets) were: Verbal Reasoning 9.34 (8.91), Physical Sciences 10.64 (10.70), Biological Sciences 11.19 (10.86); overall average of 31.17 (30.47).
The MCAT is not required for the 5 year program.

## • Number of Students Accepted to Faculty

160

## • Application Fees

$60

## • Tuition Fees

Quebec residents: $6 013.69
Out of province Canadian residents $11 357.69
International students: $24 826.01

## • Can acceptance be deferred?

Deferral is possible for the four year program, but is not probable for the five year program.

## • Province of Residence

Of the 160 students accepted, 133 will be residents of the province of Quebec. There is a possibility that 5 of the 160 are from other provinces, and the remaining 22 seats go to international students.

- ## Formula for Admissions
    The GPA is converted by the University to a score out of 5. The MCAT is also converted to a score out of five. The top students are evaluated further. The autobiographical letter and the letters of reference are each assigned a score out of 5. Currently, two one-on-one interviews are conducted and each receives a score out of 5 for a total score of 30.

    A similar formula is used for applicants from CEGEP (no MCAT).

    There are reports, unconfirmed by the Faculty, that the GPA may be adjusted by a small fraction (i.e. 0.1 - 0.3 out of 5) for students whose grades are increasing over time, whose program's difficulty is greater than the norm (including Majors, Honors), and for graduate students who expect to complete their degree prior to admission.

## What you should know about McGill University

- The Gourman Report ranks the medical school at McGill University in the category "Very Strong"; score: 4.91/5.0, currently amoung the top five in the world.
- McGill accepts the highest ratio of international students amoung Canada's medical schools.
- The five year program at McGill is for students entering directly from CEGEP studies in Quebec, most students are admitted to the four year program in which an undergraduate degree is required.
- An Early Acceptance Program exists for: (1) Quebec residents who have their CEGEP diploma (DEC) and are currently in their first year of undergraduate studies; and (2) for Canadian residents or permanent residents (landed immigrants) who are in the process of completing the second year of a four year undergraduate program. The GPA and MCAT scores tend to be significantly higher in order to gain early acceptance.
- For students who are interested in medicine as well as management, an MD/MBA program is offered at the university as well as an MD/PhD program for those interested in a career of medical research.
- Applicants from students with physical disabilities are reviewed with sympathetic consideration.
- Successful applicants are to submit a deposit of $500 to reserve their seat, this fee is then used towards tuition.
- Factors that are taken into consideration at the time of selection are: difficulty of subject matter and program studied, actual grades as well as personal characteristics and accomplishments.
- Completed graduate degrees better represent the candidate in question.
- Applications for the MD/PhD Program can be obtained from:

Program Administrator,
MD/PhD Program,
McIntyre Medical Sciences Building,
3655 Drummond Street,
Montreal, Quebec, H3G 1Y6
(514) 398-3910

• Applications for the MD/MBA Program can be obtained from:

Program Administrator
MD/MBA Program
McIntyre Medical Sciences Building
3655 Drummond Street
Montreal, Quebec, H3G 1Y6

# University of
# Ottawa

- **Address for Inquiries**

  Admissions, University of Ottawa
  Faculty of Medicine, 451 Smyth Road
  Ottawa, Ontario, Canada K1H 8M5
  (613) 562-5409; 562-5420 (FAX)
  E-mail: admissmd@uottawa.ca

- **Address for Applications**

  OMSAS
  OUAC
  Box 1328, Guelph, Ontario
  N1H 7P4; (519) 823-1940
  E-mail: omsas@netserv.ouac.on.ca
  Web site: http://www.ouac.on.ca

- **Application Deadline**

  September 15

- **Required to Submit**

  Application form and fee
  3 Confidential Assessment forms
  Autobiographical sketch (detailed)
  St. John's Ambulance and CPR or equivalent is recommended
  Interviews are held in March and May

- **Academic Requirements**

  Three years of academic work towards a bachelor's degree program must be successfully completed, as well as a full year in the following required courses: *Biochemistry, *General Chemistry, *Organic Chemistry, General Biology or Zoology, and a Humanities.    *2 of the 3 chemistry courses are required.

- **Required Academic Standing (GPA)**

  At least a B+ or a 3.3 GPA (on a 4.0 scale) is required for consideration into the program.  Students whose GPA is less than 3.4 have significantly reduced their chances for admission.  The average GPA of the 1996-97 first year medical class was 3.76/4.0.  The cutoff GPA for out-of-province students was 3.85/4.0 to gain an interview.  For the 1999-2000 and 2000-01 cycles, the cutoffs were 3.55 if your place of residence is "underserviced," 3.65 for Ottawa region or francophone, 3.83 if from elsewhere in Ontario, 3.85 if from elsewhere in the country.  The cutoffs may be adjusted somewhat from year to year.

The GPA is weighted on the last three full-time academic years according to the following: 3 times the third year, 2 times the second year, and 1 times the first year. The final figure is then divided by 6 to provide the adjusted GPA.
Admissions is based on the adjusted GPA.

- **Average MCAT Score**
  N/A

- **Number of Students Accepted to Faculty**
  123

- **Length of Program**
  4 years

- **Application Fees**
  $175 to submit your application through OMSAS, and an additional $75 is required for the university fee.

- **Tuition Fees**
  Canadian students: $10,500
  International students: $14,670

- **Can acceptance be deferred?**
  Yes, however, deferral is only granted in special circumstances.

- **Province of Residence**
  Preference is given to residents of the Ottawa region, then to those applicants of the province of Ontario, and then to candidates from the other provinces.

- **Formula for Admissions**
  The adjusted GPA accounts for 15%. Students with a satisfactory level of achievement are further evaluated. The other 85% is dependent on the interview score and assessment of the detailed Autobiographical Sketch. The other aspects of the application (i.e. Confidential Assessment Forms, etc.) serve more as 'flags'.

## What you should know about the University of Ottawa

- The Gourman Report ranks the medical school at the University of Ottawa in the category "Strong"; score: 4.51/5.0.
- All applicants must be Canadian citizens or permanent residents with the exception of children of the alumni of the University.
- All admitted applicants must undergo an interview.
- Academic excellence and interview scores are the main criteria in selection.
- No preference is given to one's program of study or university; however, the level of difficulty of courses is taken into consideration.

- Gender, race, religion nor socioeconomic status are part of the selection criterion. Preference is given to bilingual (English and French) candidates.
- The language of instruction is now available in both languages.
- A deposit of $100 is requested at the time of acceptance (conditional response) or $1000 (firm acceptance), which is deducted from tuition fees.

# NOTES

# Queen's University

- ## Address for Inquiries
  Admissions Office, Queen's University
  Faculty of Medicine, Kingston, Ontario
  Canada, K7L 3N6; (613) 533-2542; 533-3190 (FAX)
  E-mail: jeb8@post.queensu.ca
  Web site: http://meds.queensu.ca/medicine/calender/toc.html

- ## Address for Applications
  OMSAS
  OUAC
  Box 1328
  Guelph, Ontario
  N1H 7P4
  (519) 823-1940
  E-mail: omsas@netserv.ouac.on.ca
  Web site: http://www.ouac.on.ca

- ## Application Deadline
  September 15

- ## Required to Submit
  Application form and fee
  An autobiographical sketch
  3 Confidential letters of reference
  A personal identification form (five questions)
  Interviews (conducted in March)

- ## Academic Requirements
  3 full years of academic study in any university program (a minimum of 15 full courses) is required.
  Candidates are expected to have completed the following pre-requisites successfully, one full university year in:
  1) Biological sciences (e.g. botany, genetics, anatomy, biochemistry, physiology, zoology, immunology, microbiology);
  2) Physical sciences (e.g. general chemistry, physics, organic chemistry, geology);
  3) Humanities (e.g. English, French, foreign languages, film studies, religion, history, philosophy, music, drama) or
  Social Sciences (e.g. economics, sociology, geography, political science, anthropology, psychology).

- **Required Academic Standing (GPA)**

  3.62 on a 4.0 scale was the cutoff grade point average for the 2004-2005 first year class; 3.57 on a 4.0 scale was the cutoff grade point average from 1999-2000 to 2001-02. Since the cutoff is based on the median GPA of the applicant pool, it is expected to vary somewhat from year to year. If the simple average does not make it, then the average of the last 2 full-time years is compared to the cutoff.

- **Average MCAT Score**

  For the 2004-2005 first year class, the cutoffs were as follows: at least an N was attained on the Writing Sample, a 9 was the cutoff for each of Verbal Reasoning, Biological and Physical Sciences. A total sum of 32 or higher in the three multiple choice sections was needed to qualify. The 2001-02 total cutoff was 30. In a typical year, the average MCAT score of students who are accepted by the medical school is 10 - 11 per multiple choice section. Since the cutoff is based on the median MCAT scores of the applicant pool, it is expected to vary somewhat from year to year.

- **Number of Students Accepted to Faculty**

  100

- **Length of Program**

  4 years

- **Application Fees**

  $175 to submit an application through OMSAS, and an additional $75 for the university fee.

- **Tuition Fees**

  Canadian residents: $13,500

- **Can acceptance be deferred?**

  Yes, however, consideration will only be given to highly qualified applicants wishing to complete an undergraduate or graduate degree before enrolling in the Faculty.

- **Province of Residence**

  Canadians, Canadian permanent residents (landed immigrants), and children of Queen's alumni are eligible to apply. Place of residence is not a criteria in the selection of applicants.

- **Formula for Admissions**

1. GPA: the first cutoff is based on the cumulative converted grade point average of all undergraduate years or the average of the most recent two years. The current year of study is not included. [*See* Required Academic Standing]
2. MCAT Score: the second cutoff is based on the MCAT scores. The top 400 students are invited to the interview. [*See* Average MCAT Score]

3. Personal Assessment Score: candidates will be ranked for offers of admission and for placement on the waiting list based on the result of the personal assessment. There are two components to the personal assessment: (1) the Queen's autobiographical questionnaire (*"Personal Information Form"*), the autobiographical sketch, and the letters of reference account for 50% of the overall Personal Assessment Score; (2) the other 50% is based on personal interviews which are conducted over two weekends. The interview team consists of a medical student, a Faculty member and a member of the community. The interview team only has access to the autobiographical sketch.

## What you should know about Queen's University

- The Gourman Report ranks the medical school at Queen's University in the category "Very Strong"; score: 4.68/5.0.
- Program of study and level of study (i.e. undergraduate/graduate) are not criteria in the selection process at Queen's.
- The Admissions Committee seeks the following characteristics in candidates:

| Academic Abilities | Personal characteristics |
|---|---|
| commitment and achievement | ability to function as a team player |
| problem solving | ability to communicate effectively |
| critical thinking | sensitivity to the needs of others |
| self-directed learning | adaptability and ability to cope with stress |
| scientific reasoning | creativity and extracurricular activities |

- All three years of undergraduate study are considered in the selection process.
- Those whose grades and MCAT scores meet the criteria are invited for an interview. Applicants who fall just below the cutoff line have their applications reviewed by members of the Admissions committee who examine the file for unusual circumstances.
- Race, age, religion and sexual orientation are not a factor in the selection procedure.
- Place of residence is not an issue in the selection process.
- No advance standing or transfers are normally considered.
- Visit the Queen's website for an excellent description of PBL.

## NOTES

# University of Toronto

- ## Address for Inquiries
  University of Toronto, Faculty of Medicine
  Toronto, Ontario, Canada, M5S 1A8
  (416) 978-2717; 971- 2163 (FAX)
  E-mail: medicine.admiss@utoronto.ca
  Web site: http://www.library.utoronto.ca/medicine/

- ## Address for Applications
  OMSAS
  OUAC
  Box 1328
  Guelph, Ontario
  N1H 7P4
  (519) 823-1940
  E-mail: omsas@netserv.ouac.on.ca
  Web site: http://www.ouac.on.ca

- ## Application Deadline
  September 15

- ## Required to Submit
  Application form and fee
  3 Confidential Assessment Forms
  An autobiographical essay
  An autobiographical sketch
  MCAT scores
  Interviews are conducted in March and May

- ## Academic Requirements
  Applications are accepted from those who have a minimum of three full-time undergraduate years (or equivalent) or are in the process of completing their third year. University graduates from all faculties or students with 15 full course credits from any discipline are encouraged to apply. Pre-requisites for all applicants is one full year course equivalent in Humanities or Languages or Social Sciences. As well, at least two full year courses must have been completed in Life Sciences. A university course in biometrics or statistics is recommended, although not compulsory.

- ## Required Academic Standing (GPA)
  Usually 3.6 on a 4.0 scale is expected from applicants residing in Ontario.
  A minimum of 3.0/4.0 for graduate students may be acceptable.

3.7/4.0 is expected from non-Ontario applicants (3.4/4.0 for graduate students). The 2004-05 first year medical class had an adjusted average GPA of 3.82/4.0. The 1997-98 first year medical class had an adjusted average GPA of 3.84/4.0.

Entire records are used in the selection process (i.e. all three years of academic performance). However, for full-time students the GPA is adjusted by placing more weight on the applicant's best 2 years, and less weight is given to the worst year. Students who are applying during their fourth or fifth year of study have their worst year eliminated and, like other applicants, have more weight allotted to their 2 best years and less to the worst remaining year.

Specifically, for the two preceding examples, to calculate the overall adjusted academic score take 40% of each of the two best academic years and 20% of the worst academic year.

Summer courses are not considered in one's grade point average.

The current year of study will not be used to calculate your GPA to fulfill your academic requirements.

- ## Average MCAT Scores

    MCAT scores are not considered in the overall calculation for acceptance at the University of Toronto; however, low scores (below 9 in the multiple choice sections or below 'N' in the Writing Sample) may jeopardize acceptance. Thus, as a rule, MCAT scores are currently used as a 'flag'.

- ## Number of Students Accepted to Faculty

    198

- ## Length of Program

    4 Years

- ## Application Fees

    $175 to submit your application through OMSAS, and an additional $75 university fee.

- ## Tuition Fees

    Canadian residents: $15,712
    International students: $29,164

- ## Can acceptance be deferred?

    Yes

- ## Province of Residence

    No restrictions apply any longer. Traditionally, up to 35 seats were offered to out-of-province residents, 9 to international students with student visas, and up to 5 seats were available to applicants sponsored by agencies of the Government of Canada.

- ## Formula for Admissions

    The total is out of 15: a score out of 9 for the academic component and a score out of 6 for the non-academic component (i.e. 60% the former, 40% the latter).

    The academic component is composed of the adjusted GPA (*see* Required Academic Standing). The MCAT is also 'included' in this category; however, currently it is only used as a 'flag' to verify that the candidate has achieved the minimum in order to receive further evaluation. Despite the preceding, if two students have the same global score for admissions (i.e. *see the first line of this paragraph*), it is possible that the numerical score of the MCAT would be used as a tie-breaker.

    The non-academic component is composed of the autobiographical letter and sketch, and the letters of reference. The top 500 applicants are invited for interviews.

## What you should know about the University of Toronto

- The Gourman Report ranks the medical school at the University of Toronto in the category "Very Strong"; score: 4.90/5.0, currently amoung the top ten in the world.
- Applicants are rated on academic excellence, non-academic achievements and personal qualities.
- Preference is not given to any particular background of study, students from all fields of study all encouraged to apply (pre-requisites must be met however).
- Applicants from outside of Canada must complete a bachelor's degree equivalent to the one obtained in Canada.
- Applications from students who have attended a foreign medical school also may be considered granted they meet the necessary requirements.
- CEGEP applicants who wish to apply must be enrolled in 3rd year level university courses, these applicants must have at least completed a minimum of 10 courses at the time of application and must complete at least 15 full courses prior to enrollment in the Medical Faculty.
- Graduate students applying in their final stage of their program must submit an additional letter from a member of their Thesis Committee evaluating the applicants' research and stating the date in which the degree will be finalized.
- The university also offers an MD/PhD program, applications for this program must be made through OMSAS and as well an additional application that must be submitted can be obtained from:

    MD/PhD Program
    Medical Sciences Building, Room 7207
    University of Toronto
    Toronto, Ont, M5S 1A8

NOTES

# McMaster University

- ## Address for Inquiries
  Admissions and Records, HSC Room 1B7-Health
  Sciences Center, McMaster University
  1200 Main Street West, Hamilton, Ontario
  Canada L8N 3Z5; (905) 525-9140, Ext. 22235
  E-mail: mdadmit@fhs.mcmaster.ca
  Web site: http://www.fhs.mcmaster.ca/mdprog

- ## Address for Applications
  OMSAS
  OUAC
  Box 1328
  Guelph, Ontario
  N1H 7P4
  (519) 823-1940
  E-mail: omsas@netserv.ouac.on.ca
  Web site: http://www.ouac.on.ca

- ## Application Deadline
  September 15

- ## Required to Submit
  Application form and fees
  Autobiographical sketch
  1 Autobiographical Submission package
  Transcripts of all post-secondary institutions attended
  3 Confidential Assessment forms
  Interviews are conducted in March and April

- ## Academic Requirements
  Three years of undergraduate work must have been completed (in any discipline) in order to apply.
  Applicants who are applying with a CEGEP diploma must further complete 2 years of additional credit work at an accredited post-secondary institution.
  There are no other specific prerequisites required.
  Students whose first language is not English must, by the 2nd of December, provide evidence of one of the following:
  a) having received at least a score of 580 on the TOEFL (Test of English as a Foreign Language), or,
  b) proof of having attended a Canadian educational institution for at least 3 years in English, or,
  c) proof of having resided in an English-speaking country for at least four years.

- ### Required Academic Standing (GPA)
  The minimum simple average grade is B or at least 3.00.
  Students admitted to the 1995-96 first year class had the following profile: 16 students had GPAs from 3.00 to 3.29, 43 students from 3.30 to 3.59, 34 students from 3.60 to 3.89, and 7 students from 3.90 to 4.00.
  Students admitted to the 2003-2004 first year medical class had a mean GPA of approximately 3.76/4.0. The range for students admitted to the 2001-2002 class was 3.12 to 3.89.

- ### Average MCAT Score
  The MCAT is not required.

- ### Number of Students Accepted to Faculty
  138

- ### Length of Program
  3 years

- ### Application Fees
  $175 to submit your application through OMSAS, and an additional $75 university fee.

- ### Tuition Fees
  Canadian residents: $14,037
  International students: $38,970

- ### Can acceptance be deferred?
  Deferral is only permitted in exceptional cases.

- ### Province of Residence
  Priority is as follows:
  1. Northwestern Ontario and Hamilton Health Region students
  2. residents from the remaining regions of Ontario
  3. candidates from the rest of Canada (13 admitted to the 2003-2004 first year medical class).
  4. applicants from other countries.

- ### Formula for Admissions
  50% is based on the simple GPA and the other 50% is based on the autobiographical materials (i.e. McMaster's questionnaire). The top 400 students are invited for interviews.

## What you should know about McMaster University

- The Gourman Report ranks the medical school at McMaster University in the category "Very Strong"; score: 4.74/5.0.
- The problem-based learning approach to medical education, as practiced and developed at McMaster's, has served as a template for change in medical schools around the world, in the US (i.e. Harvard, Hawaii), and in Canada.
- All applicants must be proficient in the English language (*see* Academic Requirements).
- Supplementary courses are often considered, depending on the circumstances.
- Graduate work is not considered unless it is complete by the time of application. Applicants with less that a 3.0 will not be considered.
- In recent years McMaster's has had one of the highest average for age of admissions, which includes having about 15% of the class over 30 years old and a few over 40 years old.
- Transcripts from all academic institutions attended must be submitted.
- Interviews involve two components: the first being a stimulated tutorial where health problems are discussed and candidates must demonstrate their group skills and problem exploration abilities. Secondly, a personal interview is conducted. Unsuccessful applicants may re-apply the next year without prejudice (a new application form and documents must all be re-sent).
- There is no possibility of transfers or advanced standing.
- There is a possibility of being assessed under the category of "Special Applicants," for information one must contact: The MD Admissions Chair, HSC Room 1B7. One must apply in writing and submit the necessary documentation before October 1st to be considered.

# NOTES

# University of Western Ontario

- ## Address for Inquiries
  Admissions, Faculty of Medicine and Dentistry
  Medical Sciences Building
  University of Western Ontario
  London, Ontario, Canada N6A 5C1
  (519) 661-3744; 661-3797 (FAX)
  E-mail: admissions@med.uwo.ca
  Website: www.med.uwo.ca

- ## Address for Applications
  OMSAS
  OUAC
  Box 1328
  Guelph, Ontario
  N1H 7P4
  (519) 823-1940
  E-mail: omsas@netserv.ouac.on.ca
  Web site: http://www.ouac.on.ca

- ## Application Deadline
  September 15

- ## Required to Submit
  Application form and fees
  3 Confidential Assessment forms
  Autobiographical sketch
  Interviews held mostly in March
  MCAT scores
  Basic life support training

- ## Academic Requirements
  Three years of university level study are required, in any discipline.
  Prerequisites are either a full course in (a) Biology with a laboratory component; (b) a science other than Biology or Chemistry; or (c) Organic Chemistry with laboratory work.
  As well 3 full non-science courses from different disciplines are required  If an applicant does not have OAC1 high-school English or equivalent, one of the first year courses must be in English or History.
  Students applying in 2006 for entry to the 2007 first year class will likely require completion or enrolment in a full time 4 year honours program in any subject (no specific prerequisites).

- ## Required Academic Standing (GPA)
  The minimum grade point average is dependent on the number of candidates and the enrollment limitations. The minimum in 2001 was 3.60 and in 2004 the minimum was 3.70.
  Transcript marks used in the selection process are: the last year of full-time attendance and the best year of full-time undergraduate work.

- ## Average MCAT Score
  For the 2004-2005 first year medical class the minimum scores were: Verbal Reasoning 9, Physical Sciences 9, Biological Sciences 10, and the Writing Sample Q. Scores were similar for 2001-2002 with a minimum Writing Sample score of P. The minimum MCAT score is dependent on the number of candidates and the enrollment limitations and thus may vary somewhat from year to year.

- ## Number of Students Accepted to Faculty
  133

- ## Length of Program
  4 years

- ## Application Fees
  $175 to submit your application through OMSAS, and an additional $75 to apply to the University of Western Ontario.

- ## Tuition Fees
  Canadian residents: $14,795

- ## Can acceptance be deferred?
  No

- ## Province of Residence
  Canadian citizens and permanent residents (landed immigrants) need only apply. Applications will not be accepted from individuals who do not meet this criteria.

- ## Formula for Admissions
  Admission is primarily based on grades, the MCAT score and on scores received from the personal interview. Specifically, the current formula is as follows: 1/4 is based on the adjusted GPA (*see* Required Academic Standing); 1/4 is based on the MCAT (beware: UWO traditionally emphasizes the Verbal Reasoning and the Writing Sample sections); at this point, the top students as assessed from the preceding totals are invited to the interview which accounts for the final 1/2.

## What you should know about the University of Western Ontario

- The Gourman Report ranks the medical school at the University of Western Ontario in the category "Strong"; score: 4.48/5.0.
- Applicants who already possess a degree may continue to study for one additional year at the undergraduate level if they wish to improve their academic standing for their application to medical school. This special year must consist of five full courses with a minimum of four full honors courses.
- Students who are "academically competitive" may take prerequisites that they are missing in summer sessions or on a part-time basis in order to fulfill the requirements.
- Proficiency in English is a must. In fact, a composition written at the time of the interview was only recently eliminated from the admission requirements. Therefore, Verbal Reasoning and the Writing Sample (MCAT) have become important indicators of English proficiency
- Unsuccessful applicants may request a review of the Admissions Committee's decision if new and significant information is to be provided that is pertinent to the applicant's file. If an unsuccessful student wishes to re-apply the next year, they must re-submit a new application along with all the required documentation needed again.
- Transfers are only considered under very exceptional cases.
- Other programs offered are: a combined MD/PhD program, and a MD/MSc program.

## NOTES

# Northern Ontario Medical School

- ## Address for Inquiries

**Northwest Campus**
Lakehead University
955 Oliver Rd
Thunder Bay, ON
P7B 5E1
Tel: (807) 343-8100
Fax: (807) 346-7994

**Northeast Campus**
Laurentian University
935 Ramsey Lake Rd
Sudbury, ON
P3E 2C6
Tel: (705) 675-4883
Fax: (705) 675-4858

Website: http://www.normed.ca/

- ## Address for Applications
    OMSAS
    OUAC
    Box 1328
    Guelph, Ontario
    N1H 7P4
    (519) 823-1940
    E-mail: omsas@netserv.ouac.on.ca
    Web site: http://www.ouac.on.ca

- ## Application Deadline
    September 15

- ## Required to Submit
    Application form and fees
    3 Confidential Assessment forms
    Autobiographical sketch
    Interviews for selected candidates

- ## Academic Requirements

    The minimum admission requirement is a 4 year undergraduate university degree.

There are no specific course prerequisites. It is recommended that students broaden a Science degree with courses in arts, humanities and/or social sciences or an Arts degree with science courses.

- ## Required Academic Standing (GPA)

  The GPA will be determined using the marks of the last 3 years of the first 4 full-time years of undergraduate study. Graduate studies marks may be used if a GPA for graduate studies of 3.8 or greater is achieved

- ## Average MCAT Score
  The MCAT is not a requirement.

- ## Number of Students Accepted to Faculty
  56 (24 to the Thunder Bay campus and 32 to the Sudbury campus)

- ## Length of Program
  4 years

- ## Application Fees
  $175 to submit your application through OMSAS, and an additional $75 to apply to the University of Western Ontario.

- ## Tuition Fees
  To be determined.

- ## Can acceptance be deferred?
  No

- ## Province of Residence
  Canadian citizens and permanent residents (landed immigrants) need only apply. Applications will not be accepted from individuals who do not meet this criteria.

## What you should know about the Northern Ontario Medical School

- Canada's newest medical school for the whole of Northern Ontario, the Northern Ontario Medical School (NOMS) is a joint venture of Laurentian University, Sudbury and Lakehead University, Thunder Bay. With main campuses in Thunder Bay and Sudbury, NOMS will have multiple teaching and research sites distributed across Northern Ontario, including large and small communities.
- First medical class begins in September, 2005.

# University of Manitoba

- **Address for Inquiries and Applications**

  Chairman, Admissions Committee
  University of Manitoba, Faculty of Medicine
  753 McDermot Avenue, Winnipeg Manitoba
  Canada R3E 0W3; (204) 789-3569; 789-3929 (FAX)
  E-mail: med@cc.umanitoba.ca
  Website: www.umanitoba.ca/faculties/medicine/admissions/index.html

- **Application Deadline**

  October 15th

- **Required to Submit**

  Application form and fee
  An essay
  3 letters of reference
  MCAT scores
  Interview

- **Academic Requirements**

  All applicants must have attained or be in the process of completing a bachelor's degree by the end of June of the year for which admission is being sought. A full university level course must have been completed in either English or French, as well as one full course in Biochemistry. A minimum of "C" must have been attained in both of the preceding courses.

  Those with a 3 or 4 year B.A. or B.Sc., in addition to the above required courses, must have completed 2 full courses in any Humanities or Social Sciences.

  Those with a B.A. (Hons.) or a B.Sc. (Hons.), in addition to the 2 required courses, must have completed 6 credits in any of the Humanities or Social Sciences *and* as well 6 credits in any of the Physical or Natural Sciences.

  [*6 credits is equivalent to a full year course*]

  The Faculty of Medicine recommends that you take Chemistry 40 S, Physics 40 S, Math 40 S, English 40 S or French 40 S and Biology 40 S or 40 G.

- **Required Academic Standing (GPA)**

  Those who have attained an adjusted GPA of 3.60 on a 4.5 scale will be considered. Most successful applicants have adjusted GPAs in the 3.8 to 4.2 range on a 4.5 scale. The average aGPA of accepted candidates to the 2003-2004 first year class was 4.02 (3.31 for those in the Special Consideration category). Adjustments to the simple GPA are essentially made by eliminating a certain number of courses with the poorest grades, depending on the number of undergraduate courses completed.

- ## Average MCAT Score
  The overall average MCAT score for 2003-2004 was 10.37 for multiple choice sections and P for the Writing Sample. The scores ranged from 8.75 to 12.75. The minimum performance levels are as follows:
  a score of at least an "N" is expected on the Writing Sample, and a score of at least 8 is required on the 3 other sections of the MCAT. Exceptions are:
  a) an average score of 8 is attained with a 7 in one section, or
  b) an average of 8 is attained in all sections with an "M" in the Writing Sample.

- ## Number of Students Accepted to Faculty
  85

- ## Length of Program
  4 years

- ## Application Fees
  $50

- ## Tuition Fees
  $7 595

- ## Can acceptance be deferred?
  Yes

- ## Province of Residence
  Priority is given to Canadian citizens or permanent residents of Manitoba with or without a pre-medical education. Up to 7 seats may be allocated to out-of-province Canadian citizens or permanent residents.

- ## Formula for Admissions
  Based on the GPA and MCAT about 150 students are invited to the interview. The criteria for selection are as follows:

  | | | |
  |---|---|---|
  | 10% = | GPA (adjusted) |
  | 50% = | MCAT score |
  | 40% = | personal assessment score |

  Applicants' grade point averages are adjusted in a manner in which, dependent on the number of credit hours completed, a percentage of the applicant's worst marks are excluded. Students in the Special Consideration category will have the same criteria above but in the following breakdown: 10%, 20%, 70%.

## What you should know about the University of Manitoba

- The Gourman Report ranks the medical school at the University of Manitoba in the category "Strong"; score: 4.56/5.0.
- Counselling for pre-medical students is available through the Dean's office. An interview workshop is available to those who are invited to be interviewed.
- The personal assessment is based on an 800-1200 word autobiographical essay, the Writing Sample section of the MCAT, all letters from referees and by the total score achieved on the personal interview (50 - 60 minutes, audiotaped).
- A few exceptions are made for applicants who are Manitoba residents and who fall a little below expectations with regards to undergraduate achievement but who have had some sort of premedical experience. These students may apply under the "Special Consideration Category."
- Preference is given to graduates of universities in Manitoba. In 1997-98, 8 out of 70 positions went to Canadian residents from outside Manitoba. There were 4 in 2002-2003.
- No discrimination is made on the basis of race, sex, creed or national origin.
- Advanced standing is a possibility for applicants in Medicine I and II of schools that are recognized by LCME/CACMS. Advanced standing is a limited possibility for students in their second or third year of medicine who are studying at LCME accredited universities from Canada or the US.
- Applicants may wish to have their applications reconsidered, if so, they should submit a request within 10 days of the Committees decision.

## NOTES

# University of Saskatchewan

- ## Address for Inquiries and Applications
    Administrative Assistant, Admissions
    University of Saskatchewan, College of Medicine
    B 103 Health Sciences Building
    Saskatoon, Saskatchewan, Canada S7N 0W0
    (306) 966-8554; 966-6164 (FAX)
    E-mail: tokarik@amble.usask.ca
    Website: www.usask.ca/medicine

- ## Application Deadline
    December 1st: out-of-province residents
    January 15th: Saskatchewan residents

- ## Required to Submit
    Application form and fees
    1 copy of all post-secondary transcripts
    3 letters of reference
    MCAT scores
    Interview

- ## Academic Requirements
    2 years of full-time academic study are required for entry into the program of medicine, the following listed courses (University of Sasakatchewan) must be completed:
    Biology 110.6 (general)
    Chemistry 111.3 (general)
    Chemistry, Organic 251.3
    (pre-req.: Chem 111.3)
    Physics 111.6 (general)
    English 110.6 (Ontario Gr. 13 English is not considered equivalent)
    As well six credits must have been attained in Humanities or the Social Sciences.
    Biochemistry 200.3 and 211.3

    From the University of Regina, the following courses are required:
    Biology 100 and 101
    Chemistry 102 and 240
    Physics 109 and 119
    English 100 and 110
    As well, two Social Sciences or Humanities courses are necessary.
    Biochemistry 220 and 320.

    Standard First Aid certificate

- ## Required Academic Standing (GPA)
  The 2003-2004 first year medical class had an average GPA of 87.74% with a range from 81% to 94.15%. The 2002-2003 first year medical class had an average GPA of 86.75%.
  In-province students: a minimum of 78% in a two year average of full-time undergraduate study (60 credits) is required.
  Out-of-province students: a minimum of 80% average in the two best full-time undergraduate years completed at the time of application is required. In recent years, the average of the out-of-province students who were invited for interviews was 88% or higher.
  All students must have a minimum average of 70% for required courses.

- ## Average MCAT Score
  The 2003-2004 first year medical class had an average MCAT score of 9.25 in Physical Sciences, 8.67 in Verbal Reasoning and 9.25 in Biological Sciences. The MCAT minimum scores are set at 8 for multiple choice sections and N for the Writing Sample. Either one 7 or an M is acceptable.

- ## Number of Students Accepted to Faculty
  60

- ## Length of Program
  4 years

- ## Application Fees
  $40 for in-province residents
  $75 for out-of-province residents

- ## Tuition Fees
  Canadian students: $10 168

- ## Can acceptance be deferred?
  Acceptance may be deferred (usually for academic reasons).

- ## Province of Residence
  6 of the 60 seats are offered to out-of-province students who are Canadian citizens or landed immigrants who have resided in Canada for at least three years.
  3 seats are reserved for applicants of Canadian aboriginal descent.

- ## Formula for Admissions
  The average of the best two full-time undergraduate years accounts for 76%.
  The interview score accounts for the remaining 24%. In recent years, the mean interview score of students admitted to the Faculty was 21 out of 24.

## What you should know about the University of Saskatchewan

- The Gourman Report ranks the medical school at the University of Saskatchewan in the category "Strong"; score: 4.16/5.0.
- Only Canadian citizens or permanent residents are eligible to study at the University of Saskatchewan.
- Priority is given to residents of the province itself who have resided in the province for at least 3 consecutive years. Exceptions to this rule are made for members of the armed forces, for members of the RCMP, or for any family who has had to relocate due to the training or employment of a spouse.
- Aboriginal applicants require an average of 78% or above on their 2 best pre-med years. These students must also receive at least a 16 out of 24 on the personal interview. Aboriginal students shall only compete in a pool of other aboriginal students, not from the entire pool; therefore, aboriginal applicants should be sure to identify themselves on the application form.
- Summer courses are not considered in the two year average grading.
- For those who possess a graduate degree, their average can either be: (a) based on their entire undergraduate academic record and as well on the formal courses taken in their graduate faculty, or (b) based solely on their 2 best full years in their undergraduate program.
- Interviews are a crucial part in the selection process, all considered candidates are require to undergo a 45 minute interview. A score out of 24 is given for the interview.

# NOTES

# University of Alberta

- ## Address for Inquiries
    Admissions Officer, 2-45 Medical Sciences Building
    University of Alberta, Faculty of Medicine
    & Oral Health Sciences, WC Mackenzie HSC
    Edmonton, Alberta, Canada, T6G 2R7
    (780) 492-6621; 492-7303 (FAX)
    E-mail: admissions@med.ualberta.ca
    Website: www.med.ualberta.ca

- ## Address for Applications
    Office of the Registrar
    University of Alberta
    Edmonton, AB T6G 2M7

- ## Application Deadline
    November 1st

- ## Required to Submit
    Application form and fee
    An autobiographical essay
    2 letters of reference, the Faculty has specific forms
    MCAT scores
    2 copies of all post-secondary transcripts
    Interview

- ## Academic Requirements
    Most students require an undergraduate degree. Exceptional students with 2 or 3 years of full-time undergraduate study may be considered for admission.
    There are seven required courses. Five are full-year courses (6 credits): inorganic chemistry, organic chemistry, physics, biology, English; two can be half-year courses (3 credits): statistics and biochemistry.

- ## Required Academic Standing (GPA)
    For students who would have completed and undergraduate degree prior to admissions:
    In-Province: minimum GPA of 7.0 on a 9.0 scale.
    Recently, the GPA required for an interview was 7.8 on a 9.0 scale with a cumulative average of 8.43 and a prequisite average of 8.49 (2003-04).
    Out-of-Province: minimum GPA of 7.5 on a 9.0 scale (approx. 3.7/4.0).
    Recently, the GPA required for an interview was 8.0 on a 9.0 scale with an average of 8.47 (2001-02).

The current year is not included in the calculation. To convert grades to the 9.0 scale, use OMSAS' Undergraduate Grading System Conversion Table (*see* Chapter 2).

For students who have completed only two or three years of undergraduate study: minimum GPA of 8.0 on a 9.0 scale; recently, the GPA required for an interview was 8.2 on a 9.0 scale.

- **Average MCAT Score**
  10.78 (2003-04) with a minimum of "J" on the Writing Sample.
  A score of less than 7 in any section is not normally acceptable.

- **Number of Students Accepted to Faculty**
  128

- **Length of Program**
  4 years

- **Application Fees**
  $60

- **Tuition Fees**
  Canadian students: $12 066.26

- **Can acceptance be deferred?**
  Yes

- **Province of Residence**
  113 positions are offered to residents of Alberta.
  15 positions are offered to non-Alberta residents.

- **Formula for Admissions**
  The global score to rank students for admissions is derived from: the Cumulative Academic Average (*includes all academic study as a full-time student*) = 10%; the Pre-requisite GPA (*see* Required Academic Standing) = 25%; the MCAT = 15%; Writing Sample = 5%; Non-Academic Material (ie. interview, personal attributes, reference letters) = 45%.

## What you should know about the University of Alberta

- The Gourman Report ranks the medical school at the University of Alberta in the category "Strong"; score: 4.46/5.0.
- Selection is made without knowledge of applicant's race, sex, or age.
- Academic achievement, personal suitability and MCAT scores remain the basis of selection.

- For applicants who have completed four or more years of university, the Cumulative Academic Average (*see* Formula for Admissions) is calculated after deleting the worst year as long as it is neither (a) the most recent year completed nor (b) the one and only year with 5 course equivalents (i.e. 30 credits).
- Proficiency in English is required and must be demonstrated by one of the following ways:

1. Proof of 6 years of education in English, within Canada or another English speaking country, or
2. Completion of 6 full-time years of instruction or the equivalent in a Canadian school where the primary language of instruction is not English but where the level of English required for graduation, is equivalent to other Canadian educational institutions, or
3. Have attained a score of 580 of higher on the TOEFL (with a minimum of 50 on each of the three components), or at least a 90 on the MELAB (Michigan English Language Assessment Battery), or
4. Have graduated with a degree from an accredited English university, or
5. Have attained an 80% or above on Alberta English course 30 (diploma examination section only), or have received a 6 or 7 on the International Baccalaureate Higher Level English, or a score of 5 on the Advanced Placement Test course.

In addition to one of the above requirements, candidates whose native tongue is not English must take a: Test of Spoken English, and attain a score of at least 50 on the test.

- Residents of Alberta are preferred, residents are considered as those who reside in Alberta or in the Northwestern Territories or in the Yukon (for at least one continuous year).
- Early admission may be possible for those having completed 2 or 3 years in a degree program who have completed all pre-requisite work.
- Applicants of Aboriginal origin are considered separately, all native applicants are encouraged to contact the Coordinator where they can also access counseling in course selection, aid in scholastic funding, tutorial services, and help with summer employment opportunities.

Faculty of Medicine and Oral Health Sciences
Native Health-care Careers Program
2-45 Medical Sciences Building
University of Alberta
Edmonton AB T6G 2H7
(780) 492-6621

# NOTES

# University of Calgary

- ## Address for Inquiries and Applications
  Office of Admissions, University of
  Calgary, Faculty of Medicine
  3330 Hospital Drive, N.W., Calgary, Alberta
  Canada T2N 4N1; (403) 220-4262; 283-4740
  E-mail: meyers@med.ucalgary.ca
  Web site: http://www.med.ucalgary.ca/admissions

- ## Application Deadline
  Deadline for the application (web based) and fee is November 15th.
  Deadline for official transcripts, letters of reference and MCAT scores is January 15th.

- ## Required to Submit
  Application form and fee
  An employment history and list of extracurricular activities
  3 letters of reference
  An essay
  All post-secondary school transcripts
  Official MCAT score
  Personal interview

- ## Academic Requirements
  At least two full years of full-time university level study (a three year undergraduate baccalaureate degree, however, is most common).
  A pre-medical program is not required, but the following courses are recommended which are necessary for a background in medical studies:
  a full year university course in: general chemistry, general biology, organic chemistry, mammalian physiology (or comparative), biochemistry, physiology, calculus, English, physics and either psychology or sociology or anthropology.
  The Admissions Committee does consider students who have completed educational training in other disciplines for instance physical sciences, engineering, the humanities, etc...

- ## Required Academic Standing (GPA)
  The average GPA of the two best completed (at the time of application) full-time years of the entering 2002-2003 first year medical class was 3.73 on a 4.0 scale.
  Residents of Alberta must have a minimum GPA of 3.0 on a 4.0 scale when their best two completed full-time years of university are averaged.
  Out-of-province applicants must have a minimum GPA of 3.5 when their best two completed full-time years of university are averaged.
  International students must have a minimum GPA of 3.75 when their best two

completed full-time years of university are averaged.
Note: all grades are converted to the University of Calgary's 4.00 rating system.

- **Average MCAT Score**
  Students admitted to the 2002-2003 first year class had the following averages (2001-2002 in brackets): Verbal Reasoning 9.70 (9.37), Physical Sciences 10.43 (10.07), Biological Sciences 10.83 (10.25), and Writing Sample P (Q). In 2001, the average MCAT scores remained around 10-11.

- **Number of Students Accepted to Faculty**
  112

- **Length of Program**
  3 years

- **Application Fees**
  $85

- **Tuition Fees**
  Canadian students: $6 992
  International Students: $35 000.

- **Can acceptance be deferred?**
  Yes

- **Province of Residence**
  Although priority is given to applicants of Alberta, out-of-province applications are welcome. 15% of positions are available for non-Albertans, 12 positions for international students.

## What you should know about the University of Calgary

- The Gourman Report ranks the medical school at the University of Calgary in the category "Strong"; score: 4.43/5.0.
- In the criteria for selection no consideration is given to sex, religion, race or socioeconomic status.
- Any physical disabilities an applicant may experience must not interfere with the expected practices of a physician.
- Candidates from any institution who have been required to withdraw or have done so willingly, or have been expelled are not considered for admission.
- All considered applicants are invited for an hour long interview, at which time the applicant is given an additional 45 minutes to write an essay on an assigned topic.
- For unsuccessful applicants who wish to re-apply to the university, they may do so the following year without prejudice.
- A deposit of $100 is expected from accepted applicants, this deposit is later applied to

tuition fees.

- Involvement in health-care through voluntary activities or employment enhances applications, however, no weight is assigned to any specific areas of applications, all information provided is taken into consideration.

- Since the pool of applicants is so large and there are limited seats available, the Faculty of Medicine at the University of Calgary gives a high priority to non-academic qualities as all candidates in the final pool are of excellent academic standing.

- The great majority of students admitted to the Faculty have at least an undergraduate degree (1996: 65 of 69 students).

- Transfers are only considered from accredited medical schools in Canada or the US and only in special circumstances.

# University of
# British Columbia

- ## Address for Inquiries and Applications
  Office of the Dean, Faculty of Medicine
  Admissions Office, University of British
  Columbia, 317-2194 Health Sciences Mall
  Vancouver, British Columbia, Canada V6T 1Z3
  (604) 822-4482; 822-6061 (FAX)
  E-mail: admissions.md@ubc.ca
  Web site: http://www.med.ubc.ca

- ## Application Deadline
  October 1st

- ## Required to Submit
  Application form and fee
  1 copy of post secondary academic transcript
  3 letters of reference
  1 personal statement
  MCAT score report
  Personal interview may be requested

- ## Academic Requirements
  Minimum of 3 completed years in the Faculty of Science or Arts or other faculty at
  the University of British Columbia (90 credits), or the equivalent thereof. A full
  course is required in:
  - English chosen from Eng. 110, 111, 112, 120 and 121
  (English 112 recommended) or equivalent.
  - Biology 120 and 110 or 115 or 80% or better in Biology 12 or equivalent.
  - Chemistry 111 and 112 or 121 and 122 or equivalent.
  - Chemistry 203 and 204 or 231 and 232 or equivalent.
  - Biochemistry 300 or 303 or Biology 201 plus Biochemistry 302 or equivalent.

- ## Required Academic Standing (GPA)
  Minimum academic standing for admission to the Faculty of Medicine is an overall
  average of 70% (or equivalent in other grading systems). For the first year medical
  classes from 1995-96 to 2003-2004, the *average* grades of all the applicants who
  gained admission was approximately 83% from year to year.

- ## Average MCAT Score
  The 2003-2004 first year class had the following average scores by section: 9.7 (VR),
  10.6 (PS), Q (WS), 10.9 (BS).

- **Number of Students Accepted to Faculty**
  200 (256 by 2010)

- **Length of Program**
  4 years

- **Application Fees**
  BC Residents $105.00. Out-of-province applicants $155.00 plus an additional $30 for evaluation of out-of-province transcripts.

- **Tuition Fees**
  Canadian students: $14 000   (international students are not accepted)

- **Can acceptance be deferred?**
  Yes, under special circumstances deferral is a possibility for a period of one year.

- **Province of Residence**
  Preference is given to well-qualified Canadian citizens and permanent residents residing in the province of British Columbia. In 2004, 5 positions were set aside for out of province applicants.

- **Formula for Admissions**
  50% academic (transcripts and MCAT), 50% non-academic

### What you should know about the University of British Columbia

- The Gourman Report ranks the medical school at the University of British Columbia in the category "Very Strong"; score: 4.85/5.0.
- The program is growing significantly - expanding to Northern and Island campuses to, hopefully, improve access to health care in the longterm.
- Often personal interviews are conducted, in these meetings the committee is in search of students with positive personality characteristics who truly have a desire to help others, and who are extremely motivated. Other qualities sought by the committee are: demonstration of integrity, emotional stability, creativity, social concern and an ability to communicate effectively verbally as well as written.
- No particular degree is preferable during the selection process, students from all program backgrounds of study are invited to apply to UBC's Medical program.
- Complete academic records are reviewed since secondary graduation. University performance is strongly determined by a student's overall university average.
- Applicants who are successful must upon acceptance submit a deposit of $300.00 which is non-refundable, but is applied towards tuition.
- Applicants who are refused may re-apply the subsequent year without prejudice. After three unsuccessful applications, subsequent applications are generally not accepted unless followed by a five year hiatus.
- Combined BSc/MD and MD/PhD programs are available.

# Chapter 12

# DIRECTORY OF AMERICAN MEDICAL SCHOOLS

---

*To prevent disease, to relieve suffering and to heal the sick - this is our work.*

**Sir William Osler**, Aequanimitas

## The US Option

Over the years the rate of admissions to American medical schools has been consistently more than 1 in 3, while the same rate in Canada has been around 1 in 5. The grades and MCAT scores required for the average American medical school are somewhat lower as compared to the Canadian counterpart. There are several American schools that highly regard Canadian undergraduate training. Acceptance to a medical school in the US may be easier, however...

There are many serious concerns a Canadian resident must have about attending an American medical school: (i) tuition may be tens of thousands of dollars per year with little or no financial aid; (ii) attending any one of the great majority of medical schools in the US may negate any chance of returning home to practice. Either you would have to remain abroad to practice or apply to write the Canadian licencing exams, pass, and hope to get a position in an area with a little less than 24 hours sunlight in the summer!

Therefore, as a rule, if you graduate from a foreign medical school, you may have to practice medicine abroad. If you are permitted to return to Canada to practice, which is becoming increasingly difficult, it is likely that you would only be permitted a license for a rural area which has difficulty attracting doctors (i.e. North Battleford, Saskatchewan).

As for the Canadian medical schools, you should write each American school which interests you and clarify their admissions policies.

## The Medical Schools in America

*Alphabetized by State*

Office of Medical Student Services/Admissions
University of Alabama, School of Medicine
VH-100, Birmingham, Alabama
35294-0019, (205) 934-2330, 934-8724 (FAX)
Average GPA: 3.6
Average MCAT: 9.7

Office of Admissions, Rm. 2015
Medical Sciences Building, University of South Alabama
College of Medicine, Mobile, Alabama
36688-0002, (205) 460-7176, 460-6761 (FAX)
Average GPA: 3.6
Average MCAT: 9.7

Admissions Office, University of Arizona
College of Medicine, Tuscon, Arizona 85724-5075
(602) 626-6214; 626-4884 (FAX)
Average GPA: 3.5
Average MCAT: 9.4

Office of Student Admissions, Slot 551
University of Arkansas for Medical Sciences
College of Medicine, 4301 West Markam St.
Little Rock, Arkansas, 72205-7199
(501) 686-5354; 686-5873 (FAX)
Average GPA: 3.6
Average MCAT: 9.2

Admissions Office
University of California, Davis
School of Medicine, Davis, California 95616
(916) 752-2717
Average GPA: 3.5
Average MCAT: 11.0

Office of Admissions, 118 Med Surge I
UCI-College of Medicine, Irvine, California, 92717-4089
(714) 824-5388; 824-2083 (FAX); (800) 824-5388
Average GPA: 3.6
Average MCAT: 10.5

Office of Student Affairs, Division of Admissions
UCLA School of Medicine, Center for Health Sciences
Los Angeles, California, 90095-1720
(310) 825-6081
Average GPA: 3.6
Average MCAT: 10.5

Office of Admissions, 0621, Medical Teaching Facility
University of California, San Diego
School of Medicine, 9500 Gilman Drive
La Jolla, California, 92093-0621
(619) 534-3880; 534-5282 (FAX)
Average GPA: 3.6
Average MCAT: 11.0

School of Medicine, Admissions, C-200, Box 0408
University of California, San Francisco
San Francisco, California, 94143
(415) 476-4044
Average GPA: 3.7
Average MCAT: 11.0

Associate Dean for Admissions
Loma Linda University, School of Medicine
Loma Linda, California, 92350
(909) 824-4467; 824-4146 (FAX)
Average GPA: 3.6
Average MCAT: 8.9

Office of Admissions, University of Southern California
School of Medicine, 1975 Zonal Ave.
Los Angeles, California, 90033; (213) 342-2552
Average GPA: 3.5
Average MCAT: 10.0

Office of Admissions, Stanford University
School of Medicine, 851 Welch Rd., Rm. 154
Palo Alto, California, 94304-1677
(415) 723-6861; 725-4599 (FAX)
Average GPA: 3.6
Average MCAT: 10.8

Office of Admissions and Records, Box A054
University of Colorado, School of Medicine
4200 East 9th Ave., C-297, Denver, Colorado 80262
(303) 270-7361; 270-8494 (FAX)
Average GPA: 3.6
Average MCAT: 10.0


Office of Admissions and Student Affairs
University of Connecticut, School of Medicine
263 Farmington Ave., Farmington, Connecticut 06032
(203) 679-2152; 679-1282 (FAX)
Average GPA: 3.6
Average MCAT: 9.7

Office of Admissions, Yale University
School of Medicine, 367 Cedar Str.
New Haven, Connecticut, 06510
(203) 785-2643; 785-3234 (FAX)
Average GPA: 3.6
Average MCAT: 11.0

Office of Admissions, George Washington University
School of Medicine and Health Sciences
2300 Eye St., N.W., Washington, D.C., 20037
(202) 994-3506
Average GPA: 3.4
Average MCAT: 9.4

Office of Admissions, Georgetown University
School of Medicine, 3900 Reservoir Rd., N.W.
Washington, D.C., 20007; (202) 687-1154
Average GPA: 3.6
Average MCAT: 10.0

Admissions Office, Howard University
College of Medicine, 520 W St., N.W.
Washington, D.C., 20059
(202) 806-6270; 806-7934 (FAX)
Average GPA: 3.0
Average MCAT: 7.0

Chairman, Medical Selection Commitee
Box 100216, J. Hillis Miller Health Center
University of Florida, College of Medicine
Gainesville, Florida, 32610
(904) 392-4569; 392-6482 (FAX)
Average GPA: 3.4
Average MCAT: 9.4

Office of Admissions, University of Miami
School of Medicine, P.O. Box 016159
Miami, Florida, 33101
(305) 547-6791; 547-6548 (FAX); miami.md@mednet.med.miami.edu (E-mail)
Average GPA: 3.6
Average MCAT: 9.7

Office of Admissions, Box 3
University of South Florida, College of Medicine
12901 Bruce B. Downs Blvd.
Tampa, Florida, 33612-4799
(813) 974-2229; 974-4990 (FAX)
Average GPA: 3.7
Average MCAT: 9.7

Medical School Admissions, Rm. 303
Woodruff Health Sciences Center, Administration Building
Emory University, School of Medicine
Atlanta, Georgia, 30322-4510
(404) 727-5660, 727-0045 (FAX)
Average GPA: 3.7
Average MCAT: 10.2

Associate Dean for Admissions, School of Medicine
Medical College of Georgia
Augusta, Georgia, 30912-4760
(706) 721-3186; 721-0959 (FAX)
Average GPA: 3.5
Average MCAT: 9.4

Office of Admissions and Student Affairs
Mercer University, School of Medicine
Macon, Georgia, 31207
(912) 752-2542
Average GPA: 3.3
Average MCAT: 8.6

Admissions and Student Affairs

Morehouse School of Medicine
720 Westview Dr., S.W.
Atlanta, Georgia, 30310-1495
(404) 752-1650; 752-1512 (FAX)
Average GPA: 3.0
Average MCAT: 7.0

Office of Admissions, University of Hawaii
John A. Burns School of Medicine
1960 East-West Rd.
Honolulu, Hawaii, 96822
(808) 956-5446; 956-9547 (FAX)
Average GPA: 3.6
Average MCAT: 9.7

Office of the Dean of Students, University of Chicago
Pritzker School of Medicine, 924 E. 57th Street
Chicago, Illinois, 60637
(312) 702-1939; 702-2598 (FAX)
Average GPA: 3.5
Average MCAT: 10.2

Office of Admissions
UHS/Chicago Medical School, 3333 Green Bay Rd.
North Chicago, Illinois, 60064
(708) 578-3206/3207; (708) 578-3284 (FAX)
Average GPA: 3.3
Average MCAT: 9.0

Office of Medical College Admissions
Rm. 165 CME M/C 783, University of Illinois
College of Medicine, 808 S. Wood St.
Chicago, Illinois, 60612, (312) 996-5635; (312) 996-6693 (FAX)
Average GPA: 3.4
Average MCAT: 9.3

Office of Admissions, Rm. 1752
Loyola University Medical Center, Stritch School of Medicine
2160 South First Ave., Maywood, Illinois, 60153
(708) 216-3229
Average GPA: 3.5
Average MCAT: 9.5

Associate Dean for Admissions

Northwestern University Medical School
303 East Chicago Ave., Chicago, Illinois 60611
(312) 503-8206
Average GPA: 3.6
Average MCAT: 9.7

Office of Admissions, 524 Academic Facility
Rush Medical College of Rush University
600 South Paulina St., Chicago, Illinois
60612, (312) 942-6913; 942-2333 (FAX)
Average GPA: 3.4
Average MCAT: 9.1

Office of Student and Alumni Affairs
Southern Illinois University, School of Medicine, P.O. Box 19230
Springfield, Illinois, 62794-9230
(217) 524-0326; (217) 785-5538 (FAX)
Average GPA: 3.5
Average MCAT: 8.8

Medical School Admissions Office
Fesler Hall 213, Indiana University, School of Medicine, 120 South Dr.
Indianapolis, Indiana, 46202-5113
(317) 274-3772
Average GPA: 3.7
Average MCAT: 9.7

Director of Admissions, 100 CMAB
University of Iowa, College of Medicine
Iowa City, Iowa, 52242-1101
(319) 335-8052; 335-8049 (FAX)
Average GPA: 3.6
Average MCAT: 9.5

Associate Dean for Admissions
University of Kansas, School of Medicine
3901 Rainbow Blvd., Kansas City, Kansas 66160-7301
(913) 588-5245; 588-5259
Average GPA: 3.6
Average MCAT: 9.1

Admissions, Rm. MN-104, Office of Education

University of Kentucky College of Medicine, Chandler Medical Center, 800 Rose St.
Lexington, Kentucky, 40536-0084
(606) 323-6161; 323-2076 (FAX)
Average GPA: 3.6
Average MCAT: 9.0

Office of Admissions, School of Medicine
Health Sciences Center, University of Louisville
Louisville, Kentucky, 40292; (502) 852-5193
Average GPA: 3.4
Average MCAT: 8.9

Admissions Office, Louisiana State University
School of Medicine in New Orleans
1901 Perdido Street, New Orleans, Louisiana
70112-1393; (504) 568-6262; 568-7701 (FAX)
Average GPA: 3.4
Average MCAT: 8.6

Office of Student Admissions, Louisiana State University
Medical Center, School of Medicine in Shreveport
P.O.Box 33932, Shreveport, Louisiana, 71130-3932
(318) 674-5190; 674-5244 (FAX)
Average GPA: 3.5
Average MCAT: 8.8

Office of Admissions, Tulane School of Medicine
1430 Tulane Avenue, New Orleans, Louisiana, 70112-2699
(504) 588-5187
Average GPA: 3.5
Average MCAT: 9.5

Committee on Admission, Johns Hopkins University
720 Rutland Avenue, Baltimore
Maryland 21205-2196; (410) 955-3182; http://infonet.welch.jhu.edu (Internet)
Average GPA: 3.7
Average MCAT: 11.0

Committee on Admissions, Room 1-005
University of Maryland, School of Medicine
655 West Baltimore Street, Baltimore, Maryland
(410) 706-7478
Average GPA: 3.6
Average MCAT: 9.0

Admissions Office, Room A-1041

Uniformed Services University of the Health Sciences
F. Edward Hebert School of Medicine, 4301 Jones Bridge Road
Bethesda, Maryland, 20814-4799
(301) 295-3101; 295-3545 (FAX);(800) 772-1743
Average GPA: 3.5
Average MCAT: 10.2

Admissions Office, Building L, Room 124,
Boston University School of Medicine
80 East Concord Street, Boston
Massachusetts 02118; (617) 638-4630
Average GPA: 3.3
Average MCAT: 9.1

Administrator of Admissions, Harvard Medical School
25 Shattuck Street, Building A-210, Boston
Massachusetts 02115-6092
(617) 432-1550; 432-3307 (FAX)
Average GPA: 3.7
Average MCAT: 11.0

Associate Dean for Admissions
University of Massachusetts Medical School
55 Lake Avenue, North Worcester
Massachusetts 01655; (508) 856-2323
Average GPA: 3.5
Average MCAT: 10.0

Office of Admissions, Tufts University School
of Medicine, 136 Harrison Avenue, Stearns 1
Boston, Massachusetts 02111; (617) 636-6571
Average GPA: 3.5
Average MCAT: 9.2

College Human Medicine, Office of Admissions
A-239 Life Sciences, Michigan State University, East Lansing, Michigan 48824-
1317 (517) 353-9620; (517) 432-1051 (FAX); MDAdmissions@msu.edu (E-
mail)
Average GPA: 3.4
Average MCAT: 9.3

Admissions Office, M4130 Medical Science I Building
University of Michigan Medical School
Ann Arbor, Michigan 48109-0611
(313) 764-6317; 936-3510 (FAX)
Average GPA: 3.7
Average MCAT: 10.7

Director of Admissions, Wayne State University
School of Medicine, 540 East Canfield
Detroit, Michigan 48201; (313) 577-1466
Average GPA: 3.5
Average MCAT: 8.9

Admissions Committee, Mayo Medical School
200 First Street, S.W., Rochester,
Minnesota 55905; (507) 284-3671; 284-2634 (FAX)
Average GPA: 3.7
Average MCAT: 10.0

Office of Admissions, Room 107
University of Minnesota-Duluth
School of Medicine, 10 University Drive
Duluth, Minnesota 55812
(218) 726-8511; (218) 726-6235 (FAX)
Average GPA: 3.5
Average MCAT: 10.0

Office of Admissions and Student Affairs
Box 293-UMHC, University of Minnesota Medical School
420 Delaware Street, S.E., Minneapolis,
Minnesota 55455-0310; (612) 624-1122; 626-6800 (FAX)
Average GPA: 3.6
Average MCAT: 9.7

Chairman, Admissions Committee
University of Mississippi, School of Medicine
2500 North State Street, Jackson
Mississippi 39216-4505; (601) 984-5010; 984-5008 (FAX)
Average GPA: 3.6
Average MCAT: 9.0

Office of Admissions, MA202 Medical Sciences Building
University of Missouri-Columbia, School of Medicine
One Hospital Drive, Columbia
Missouri 65212; (314) 882-2923; 884-4808 (FAX)
Average GPA: 3.7
Average MCAT: 9.3

Council on Selection, University of
Missouri-Kansas City, School of Medicine
2411 Holmes, Kansas City,
Missouri 64108; (816) 235-1870; 235-5277 (FAX)
Average GPA: 3.0
Average MCAT: 8.0

Nancy McPeters, Admissions Committee
Saint Louis University, School of Medicine
1402 South Grand Boulevard, St.Louis
Missouri 63104; (314) 577-8205; 577-8214 (FAX)
Average GPA: 3.7
Average MCAT: 10.4

Office of Admissions, Washington University
School of Medicine, 660 South Euclid Avenue #8107
St.Louis, Missouri 63110;
(314) 362-6857; 362-4658 (FAX)
Average GPA: 3.8
Average MCAT: 11.4

Medical School Admissions Office
Creighton University, 2500 California Plaza
Omaha, Nebraska 68178; (402) 280-2798; (402) 280-1241 (fax)
Average GPA: 3.6
Average MCAT: 8.8

Office of Academic Affairs, Room 4004
University of Nebraska College of Medicine
Conkling Hall, 600 South 42nd Street,
Omaha, Nebraska 68198-4430
(402) 559-4205; 559-4104 (FAX)
Average GPA: 3.8
Average MCAT: 9.2

Office of Admissions and Student Affairs
University of Nevada, School of Medicine, mail stop 357
Reno, Nevada 89557
(702) 784-6063; 784-6096 (FAX)
Average GPA: 3.6
Average MCAT: 9.3

Office of Admissions, Dartmouth Medical School
7020 Remsen, Rm.306, Hanover, New Hampshire
03755-3833, (603) 650-1505; 650-1614 (FAX)
Average GPA: 3.5
Average MCAT: 9.6

Director of Admissions
UMDNJ-New Jersey Medical School, 185 South Orange Avenue
Newark, New Jersey 07103;
(201) 982-4631; (201) 982-7986 (FAX)
Average GPA: 3.4
Average MCAT: 9.6

Office of Admissions
UMDNJ-Robert Wood Johnson Medical School
675 Hoes Lane, Piscataway, New Jersey 08854-5635
(908) 235-4576; (908) 235-5078 (FAX)
Average GPA: 3.5
Average MCAT: 9.6

Office of Admissions, Basic Medical Sciences Building
Room 107, University of New Mexico, School of Medicine
Albuquerque, New Mexico 87131-5166
(505) 277-4766; 277-2755 (FAX)
Average GPA: 3.5
Average MCAT: 8.8

Office of Admissions, A-3, Albany Medical College
47 New Scotland Avenue, Albany
New York 12208; (518) 262-5521; (518) 262-5887 (FAX)
Average GPA: 3.4
Average MCAT: 9.9

Office of Admissions, Albert Einstein College of
Medicine of Yeshiva University, Jack and Pearl
Resnick Campus, 1300 Morris Park Avenue, Bronx, New York 10461
(718) 430-2106, (718) 430-8825 (FAX); admissions@aecom.yu.edu (E-mail)
Average GPA: 3.7
Average MCAT: 10.0

Columbia University, College of Physicians
and Surgeons, Admissions Office, Room 1-416
630 West 168th Street, New York,
New York 10032; (212) 305-3595
Average GPA: 3.5
Average MCAT: 10.7

Office of Admissions, Cornell University
Medical College, 445 East 69th Street
New York, New York 10021; (212) 746-1067
Average GPA: 3.6
Average MCAT: 10.6

Office for Admissions, Mount Sinai School of
Medicine, Annenberg Building, Room 5-04
One Gustave L.Levy Place-Box 1002
New York, New York 10029-6574
(212) 241-6696
Average GPA: 3.52
Average MCAT: 10.2

Office of Admissions, Room 127
Sunshine Cottage, New York Medical College
Valhalla, New York 10595
(914) 993-4507
Average GPA: 3.3
Average MCAT: 10.0

Office of Admissions, New York University
School of Medicine, P.O. Box 1924
New York, New York 10016; (212) 263-5290
Average GPA: 3.6
Average MCAT: 10.7

Director of Admissions, University of Rochester
School of Medicine and Dentistry, Medical
Center Box 601, Rochester, New York 14642
(716) 275-4539; 273-1016 (FAX)
Average GPA: 3.6
Average MCAT: 10.0

Director of Admissions, State University of
New York, Health Science Center at Brooklyn, 450 Clarkson Avenue-Box 60M
Brooklyn, New York 11203; (718) 270-2446
Average GPA: 3.5
Average MCAT: 9.3

Office of Medical Admissions, State University of
New York at Buffalo, CFS Building, Room 35
Buffalo, New York 14214-3013; (716) 829-3465
Average GPA: 3.7
Average MCAT: 10.4

Committee on Admissions, Level 4, Room 147
Health Sciences Center, SUNY at Stony Brook
School of Medicine, Stony Brook, New York
11794-8434; (516) 444-2113, 444-2202 (FAX)
Average GPA: 3.5
Average MCAT: 10.5

Admissions Committee, State University of
New York, Health Science Center at Syracuse
College of Medicine, 155 Elizabeth Blackwell Street
Syracuse, New York 13210; (315) 464-4570; 464-8867 (FAX)
Average GPA: 3.5
Average MCAT: 9.1

Office of Medical School Admissions

Bowman Gray School of Medicine of Wake
Forest University, Medical Center Boulevard,
Winston-Salem, North Carolina 27157-1090
(919) 716-4264; 716-5807 (FAX)
Average GPA: 3.4
Average MCAT: 9.7

Committee on Admissions, Duke University
School of Medicine, Duke University Medical Center
P.O. Box 3710; Durham, North Carolina 27710
(919) 684-2985; 684-8893 (FAX)
Average GPA: 3.6
Average MCAT: 10.8

Associate Dean, Office of Admissions
East Carolina University, School of Medicine
Greenville, North Carolina 27858-4354; (919) 816-2202
Average GPA: 3.5
Average MCAT: 8.5

Admissions Office, CB# 7000 MacNider Hall
University of North Carolina at Chapel Hill, School of Medicine, Chapel Hill
North Carolina 27599-7000; (919) 962-8331
Average GPA: 3.4
Average MCAT: 9.0

Secretary, Committee on Admissions
University of North Dakota, School of Medicine
501 North Columbia Road, Grand Forks
North Dakota 58202-9037; (701) 777-4221; 777-4942 (FAX)
Average GPA: 3.6
Average MCAT: 8.7

Associate Dean for Admissions and Student Affairs
Case Western Reserve University, School of Medicine
10900 Euclid Ave., Cleveland, Ohio 44106-4920
(216) 368-3450; 368-4621 (FAX)
Average GPA: 3.5
Average MCAT: 10.0

Office of Admissions, Room E-251, MSB
ML#552, University of Cincinnati
College of Medicine, 231 Bethesda Avenue, P.O. Box 670552
Cincinnati, Ohio 45267-0552
(513) 558-7314; 558-1165 (FAX)
Average GPA: 3.5
Average MCAT: 9.5

Admissions Office, Medical College of Ohio
P.O. Box 10008, Toledo, Ohio 43699
(419) 381-4229; 381-4005 (FAX)
Average GPA: 3.48
Average MCAT: 9.17

Office of Admissions and Educational Research
North Eastern Ohio Universities
College of Medicine, P.O.Box 95
Rootstown, Ohio 44272-0095; (216) 325-2511
Average GPA: 3.6
Average MCAT: 9.1

Admissions Committee, 270-A Meiling Hall
Ohio State University, College of Medicine
370 West Ninth Avenue, Columbus, Ohio 43210-1238
(614) 292-7137; 292-1544 (FAX)
Average GPA: 3.5
Average MCAT: 10.0

Office of Student Affairs/Admissions
Wright State University, School of Medicine
P.O.Box 1751, Dayton, Ohio 45401
(513) 873-2934; 873-3322 (FAX)
Average GPA: 3.5
Average MCAT: 8.0

Susan Masara, Director for Student Affairs
University of Oklahoma, College of Medicine, P.O.Box 26901
Oklahoma City, Oklahoma 73190; (405) 271-2331; 271-3032 (FAX)
Average GPA: 3.6
Average MCAT: 9.44

Office of Education and Student Affairs, L102
Oregon Health Sciences University
3181 S. W. Sam Jackson Park Road, Portland
Oregon 97201; (503) 494-4499; 494-3400 (FAX)
Average GPA: 3.6
Average MCAT: 9.9

Medical School Admissions, Mail Stop 442
Hahnemann University, School of Medicine
Broad and Vine Streets, Philadelphia
Pennsylvania 19102-1192; (215) 762-7600; 762-8654 (FAX)
Average GPA: 3.5
Average MCAT: -

Associate Dean for Admissions, Jefferson
Medical College of Thomas Jefferson University
1025 Walnut Street, Philadelphia
Pennsylvania 19107; (215) 955-6983; (215) 923-6939 (FAX)
Average GPA: 3.5
Average MCAT: 9.9

Associate Dean for Student Affairs (Admissions)
Medical College of Pennsylvania, 2900 Queen Lane
Avenue, Philadelphia, Pennsylvania 19129
(215) 991-8202; (215) 843-1766 (FAX)
Average GPA: 3.6
Average MCAT: 11.0

Office of Student Affairs, Pennsylvania State
University, College of Medicine, P.O.Box 850
Hershey, Pennsylvania 17033; (717) 531-8755; (717) 531-6225 (FAX)
Average GPA: 3.7
Average MCAT: 9.1

Director of Admissions and Financial Aid
Edward J.Stemmler Hall, Suite 100, University of Pennsylvania, School of
Medicine
Philadelphia, Pennsylvania 19104-6056
(215) 898-8001; 898-0833 (FAX)
Average GPA: -
Average MCAT: -

Office of Admissions, 518 Scaife Hall
University of Pittsburgh, School of Medicine
Pittsburgh, Pennsylvania 15261; (412) 648-9891; 648-8768 (FAX)
Average GPA: 3.6
Average MCAT: 10.7

Admissions Office, Suite 305, Student
Faculty Center, Temple University
School of Medicine, Broad and Ontario Streets
Philadelphia, Pennsylvania 19140
(215) 707-3656; (215) 707-6932 (FAX)
Average GPA: 3.4
Average MCAT: 10.0

Office of Admissions, Universidad Central
del Caribe, School of Medicine, Ramon Ruiz
Arnau University Hospital, Call Box 60-327
Bayamon, Puerto Rico 00960-6032
(809) 740-1611 Ext.210; 269-7550 (FAX)
Average GPA: 3.1
Average MCAT: 6.0

Admissions Office, Ponce School of Medicine
P.O.Box 7004, Ponce, Puerto Rico  00732
(809) 840-2511; (809) 751-3284 (FAX)
Average GPA: 3.3
Average MCAT: 6.1

Central Admissions Office, School of Medicine
Medical Sciences Campus, University of Puerto Rico
P.O.Box 365067, San Juan, Puerto Rico 00936-5067
(809) 758-2525, Ext. 5213
Average GPA: 3.6
Average MCAT: 7.5

Office of Admissions
Brown University School of Medicine, 97 Waterman St., Box GA 212
Providence, Rhode Island 02912-9706
(401) 863-2149; 863-2660 (FAX)
Average GPA: 3.4
Average MCAT: N/A

University Registrar and Director of Admissions
Medical University of South Carolina
171 Ashley Avenue, Charleston, South Carolina
29425; (803) 792-3281; 792-3764 (FAX)
Average GPA: 3.4
Average MCAT: 9.0

Associate Dean for Student Programs
University of South Carolina, School
of Medicine, Columbia, South Carolina 29208
(803) 733-3325; 733-3328 (FAX)
Average GPA: 3.4
Average MCAT: 9.0

Office of Student Affairs, Room 105
University of South Dakota, School of
Medicine, 414 East Clark Street
Vermillion, South Dakota 57069-2390
(605) 677-5233; 677-5109 (FAX)
Average GPA: 3.6
Average MCAT: 8.4

Assistant Dean for Admissions and Records
East Tennessee State University, James H.
Quillen College of Medicine, P.O.Box 70580
Johnson City, Tennessee 37614-0580
(615) 929-6221; 461-7040 (FAX)
Average GPA: 3.3
Average MCAT: 9.1

Director, Admissions and Records
Meharry Medical College, School of Medicine
1005 D.B.Todd, Jr. Boulevard, Nashville
Tennessee 37208; (615) 327-6223; 327-6228 (FAX)
Average GPA: 3.1
Average MCAT: 7.5

University of Tennessee, Memphis
College of Medicine, 790 Madison Avenue
Memphis, Tennessee 38163-2166; (901) 448-5559
Average GPA: 3.5
Average MCAT: 9.5

Office of Admissions, 209 Light Hall
Vanderbilt University, School of Medicine
Nashville, Tennessee 37232-0685
(615) 322-2145; 343-8397 (FAX)
Average GPA: 3.8
Average MCAT: 11.2

Office of Admissions, Baylor College of
Medicine, One Baylor Plaza, Houston
Texas 77030; (713) 798-4841
Average GPA: 3.7
Average MCAT: 11.0

Associate Dean for Student Affairs and Admissions,
Texas A&M University College of Medicine, College Station
Texas 77843-1114; (409) 845-7744, 847-8663 (FAX)
Average GPA: 3.6
Average MCAT: 9.3

Office of Admissions, Texas Tech University
Health Sciences Center, School of Medicine
Lubbock, Texas 79430; (806) 743-3005
743-3021 (FAX)
Average GPA: 3.6
Average MCAT: 8.8

Office of the Registrar, University of Texas
Southwestern Medical Center at Dallas
5323 Harry Hines Boulevard, Dallas, Texas
75235-9096; (214) 648-2670; 648-3289 (FAX)
Average GPA: 3.6
Average MCAT: 10.3

Office of Admissions, G.210, Ashbel Smith Building
University of Texas Medical Branch at Galveston
School of Medicine, Galveston, Texas 77555-1317
(409) 772-3517; 772-5753 (FAX)
Average GPA: 3.5
Average MCAT: 9.3

Office of Admissions-Room G-024
University of Texas, Medical School at
Houston, P.O.Box 20708, Houston
Texas 77225; (713) 792-4711; 794-4238 (FAX)
Average GPA: 3.5
Average MCAT: 8.7

Medical School Admissions, Registrar's Office
University of Texas, Health Science Center at
San Antonio, 7703 Floyd Curl Dr., San Antonio
Texas 78284-7701; (210) 567-2665; (210) 567-2685 (FAX)
Average GPA: 3.5
Average MCAT: 9.3

Millie M. Peterson, Director, Medical School
Admissions, University of Utah, School of Medicine, 50 North Medical Drive
Salt Lake City, Utah 84132; (801) 581-7498; 585-3300 (FAX)
Average GPA: 3.5
Average MCAT: 10.5

Admissions Office, E-109 Given Building
University of Vermont, College of Medicine
Burlington, Vermont 05405
(802) 656-2154; 656-8577 (FAX)
Average GPA: 3.4
Average MCAT: 9.0

Office of Admissions, Eastern Virginia Medical
School, 700 Olney Road, Norfolk
Virginia 23507-1696
(804) 446-5812; 446-5817 (FAX)
Average GPA: 3.3
Average MCAT: 9.0

Medical School Admissions, Virginia Commonwealth
University, Medical College of Virginia
MCV Station, Box 980565, Richmond, Virginia
23298-0565; (804) 828-9629, 828-7628 (FAX)
Average GPA: 3.4
Average MCAT: 9.9

Medical School Admissions Office, Box 235
University of Virginia, School of Medicine
Charlottesville, Virginia 22908
(804) 924-5571; 982-2586 (FAX)
Average GPA: 3.6
Average MCAT: 10.3

Admissions Office (SC-64), Health Sciences
Center A-300, University of Washington
Seattle, Washington 98195; (206) 543-7212
Average GPA: 3.5
Average MCAT: 10.1

Admissions Office, Marshall University
School of Medicine, 1542 Spring Valley Drive
Huntington, West Virginia 25755
(304) 696-7312; (800) 544-8514
Average GPA: 3.4
Average MCAT: 8.2

Office of Admissions and Records
West Virginia University, Health Sciences
Center, P.O. Box 9815, Morgantown, West Virginia
26506; (304) 293-3521, 293-4973 (FAX)
Average GPA: 3.6
Average MCAT: 9.0

Office and Admissions and Registrar
Medical College of Wisconsin
8701 Watertown Plank Road, Milwaukee
Wisconsin 53226; (414) 456-8246
Average GPA: 3.6
Average MCAT: 9.5

Admissions Committee, Medical Sciences Center
Room 1205, University of Wisconsin Medical
School, 1300 University Avenue, Madison
Wisconsin 53706; (608) 263-4925; 262-2327 (FAX)
Average GPA: 3.6
Average MCAT: 9.5

# Appendix

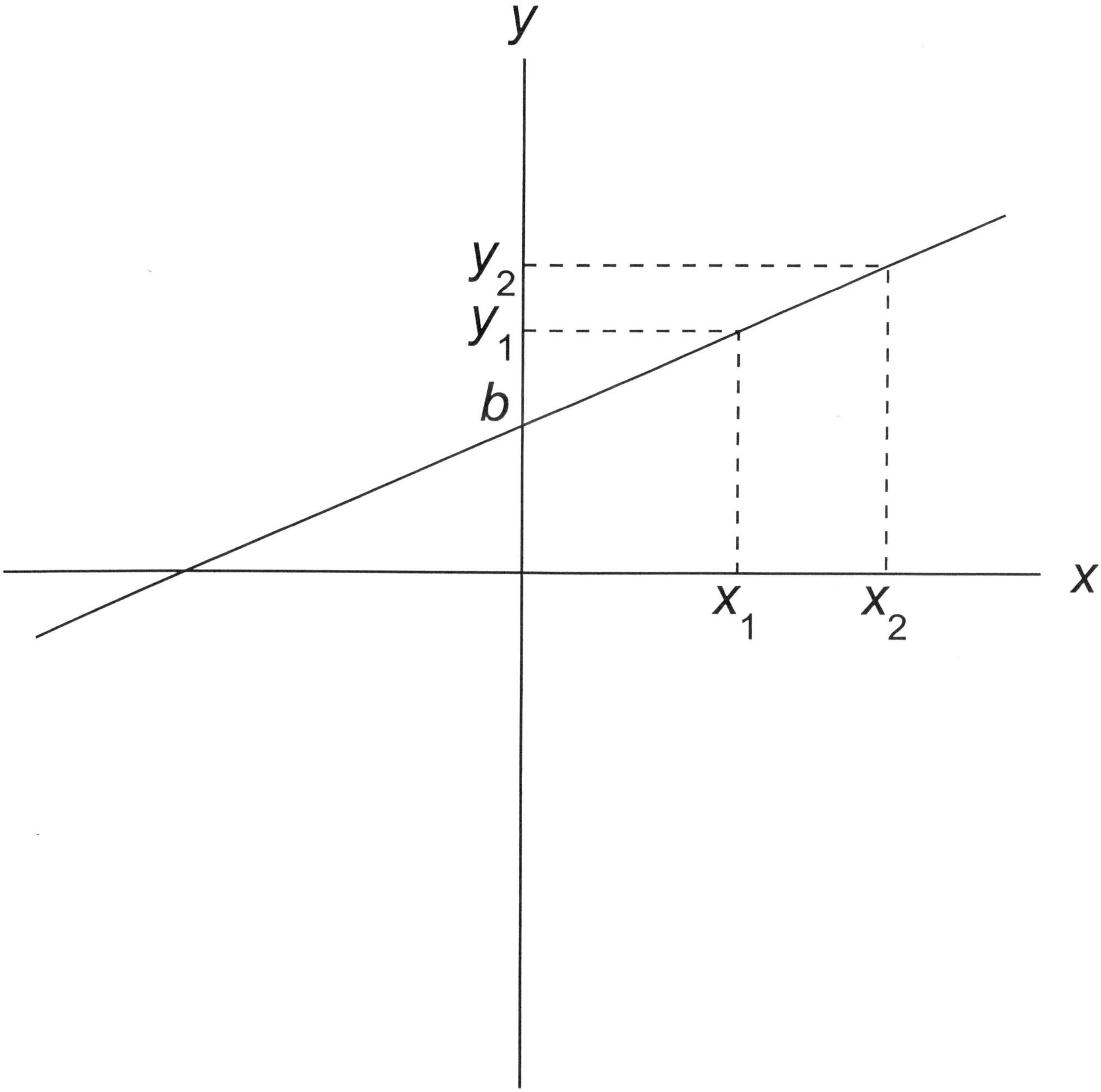

y
$y_2$
$y_1$
b
x
$x_1$
$x_2$

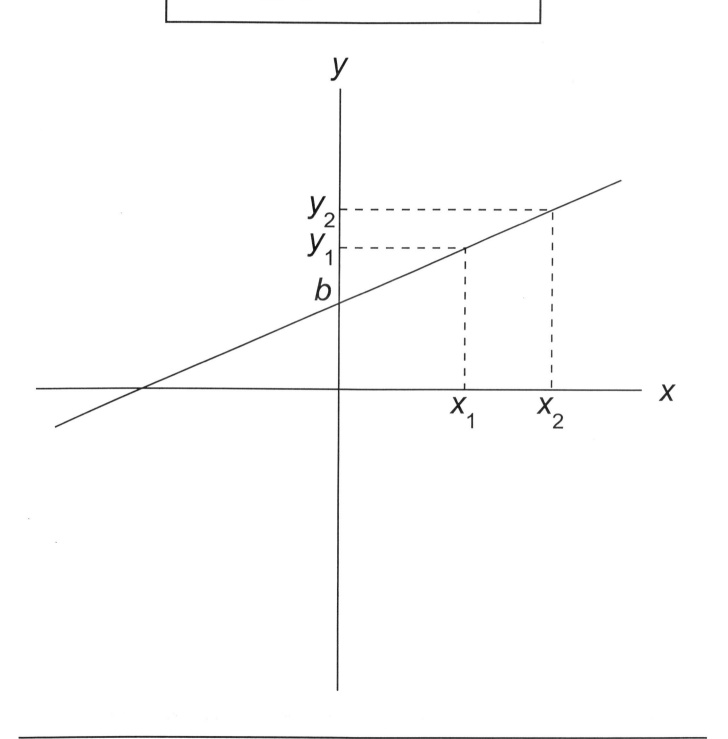

# Appendix A

# THE HIPPOCRATIC OATH

Now being admitted to the profession of medicine,
I solemnly pledge to consecrate my life to the service of humanity.
I will give respect and gratitude to my deserving teachers
and in my turn I will teach and I will study.
I will practice medicine with conscience and dignity.
The health and life of my patients will be my first consideration.
I will hold in confidence all that my patient confides in me.

I will maintain the honor and the noble traditions
of the medical profession.
I will not permit consideration of race, religion, nationality,
ideology, or social standing to intervene
between my duty and my patient.

I will maintain the utmost respect for human life. Even under threat, I will not
use my knowledge contrary to the laws of humanity.

These promises I make freely and upon my honor.

[*modified Geneva version*]

# Appendix B

# STUDY AIDS FOR THE MCAT

## B.1 Study Aids

Many students use The Gold Standard and the AAMC materials as the cornerstone to their MCAT preparation. Some students seek adjuncts to their preparation. This appendix is for those students.

## B.2 MCAT Video CD-ROMs

These 16 videos, written and edited by Dr. Ferdinand, contain explanations to all the science subjects that you are responsible for learning in order to master the MCAT. Furthermore, each "seminar" is cross-referenced to the current edition of The Gold Standard. Also included are equation lists to memorize, organic chemistry reaction summaries, and tips, questions and answers which are different than those included in The Gold Standard. The CD's can be played on a regular personal computer (PC). Avoid using these videos for cramming! They are available at participating bookstores or at MCAT-prep.com.

## B.3 The Silver Bullet Audio Cassettes

The Silver Bullet Audio Cassettes contain approximately four hours of recorded science information. Reviews of the three science subjects - Chemistry, Physics and Biology - range from 1 to 2 hours for each topic. The information on the cassettes was provided from Dr. Ferdinand's condensed notes.

The cassettes are not meant as a source to take notes from since the information is already in The Gold Standard. Rather, the cassettes are used as a source of repetition (i.e. in a car stereo or walkman on the way to work, school, etc.). Your friends may be listening to Mick Jagger or Michael Jackson but you can be listening to $F = ma$ or $PV = nRT$, and when you think about it... that's cool! These cassettes are available at participating bookstores or at MCAT-prep.com, amazon.com and futuredoctor.net.

## B.4 The Gold Standard - MCAT

The only source that a student needs for a science review for the MCAT is present in The Gold Standard - MCAT. It is comprehensive, complete and it is easy to read and study from. Sample pull-out exams are included. It is available at your local university bookstore, Chapters, or at the bookstore at MCAT-prep.com, chapters.ca and futuredoctor.net.

## B.5 The Toronto MCAT Clinic

Every summer in the month of July or August, Dr. Ferdinand travels to Toronto and runs an "MCAT Clinic" for one week. The Clinic is 6 hours/day Monday to Friday, and 9 hours/day Saturday and Sunday. The week includes a science review, MCAT problem solving sessions, and the writing of a full length practice exam which is corrected and returned to students on the same day. For information regarding registration and accommodations, or for online MCAT courses, get on the Net at www.prep.com or MCAT-prep.com.

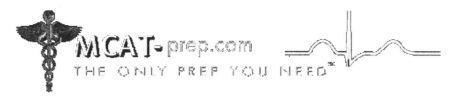

**To All Pre-Med Students, are _YOU_ preparing for the MCAT? Yes, then look no further. We are the leaders in MCAT preparation with the most comprehensive and the most complete materials that you will need to prepare YOU for the MCAT.**

## The _Updated_ Black Book
## on Canadian Medical Schools.

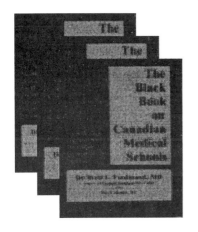

- Contains **everything** you need to know about each Canadian medical school.
- Also included: **Directory** of all US medical schools including average **GPAs** and **MCAT** scores of admitted students.
- **Do's** and **Don'ts** for the medical school interview, etc.
- A **must** have resource for all Pre-Med students.
- **Complete** information compiled in one book.

## The _NEW 2004-2005_ Gold Standard
## For Medical School Admissions

- The _most complete_ MCAT text ever written.
- Covers _all aspects_ of medical school admissions.
- Includes a comprehensive and easy to understand _review_ of the MCAT, 4 full-length _practice exams_ with explanations.
- 10 years and still _#1 in Canada_.

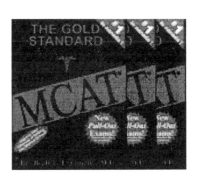

---

**Available at your local university bookstore and participating Chapters.**

---

## WEB SITE : WWW.MCAT-Prep.com

**The one place to go for all your MCAT materials and information.**

| | | |
|---|---|---|
| Books & Materials | Video CD ROMs | Audio Cassettes |
| Live Seminars | Virtual Classrooms | Interactive tools |

**SPECIAL OFFER : <u>Save 35%</u>** on the Platinum Program which consists of Video CD-ROMs, chat rooms, live online teaching, audio cassettes, online and paper exams including all released **actual past MCAT exams**, message boards, comprehensive review books and interactive programs including a speed reading program. Consult www.MCAT-Prep.com for more information and offers.